It's a Vet's Life

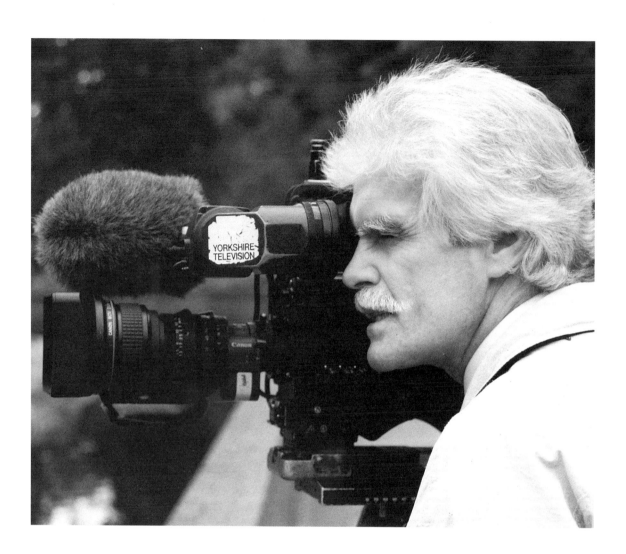

It's a Vet's Life

The Story of Television Vet
John Baxter

BⒺXTREE

Acknowledgements

This book is dedicated to my wife, Alice, who truly believed that it would never be written, to my surgery staff, the B Team, for all their support in my busy life, and not least to my many friends at Yorkshire Television for all their expert help and kindness in my years on the box.

Photograph Acknowledgements

My love of photography makes me appreciate all the more, the many talents of my nurse Bernie, who took most of the medical pictures in this book. I must also express my gratitude to the many stills photographers at Yorkshire Television and in particular to Charlie Flynn, who not only filmed 'It's a Vet's Life' as cameraman/director, but found time to take many of the publicity shots. Finally, I am indebted to my son, Lindsay, who produced the front cover photograph, and took several of the more personal shots.

First published in Great Britain in 1995 by Boxtree Limited

Text © John Baxter 1995

Designed by Behram Kapadia

Printed and bound in Bath by The Bath Press for

Boxtree Limited
Broadwall House
21 Broadwall
London SE1 9PL

A CIP catalogue entry for this book is available from the British Library.

ISBN 1 85283 942 2

Contents

Chapter 1

In the Beginning

As long as I can remember, I have found all living things incredibly fascinating. So for me, the second youngest in a family of eleven, living in a poor mining town in Fife, it was a day to remember when I was given the 'once-in-a-lifetime' chance of visiting Edinburgh Zoo. From the impressive size of the gigantic African elephants to the latent threat of the salamander lying motionless in its private pool, I was enthralled.

In the chattering, smelly monkey house, I learned much about myself and about man's closest ancestor. In the sad eyes of the great orang-utan, as he sat bored in his cage of concrete and steel, I learned something of man's inhumanity to more than man. Although I drank in many of the wonders of the wild animal world held captive in this windy Scottish capital, I could never shake off the feeling that it was man's selfishness that had brought them here and that this was Nature at its most unnatural.

The cheeky Scottish sparrows in their drab brown plumage had a perky air of superiority, as they freely pecked for titbits among the more exotically feathered captives from far-off lands. The Mallard ducks, who stopped off for some easy pickings in the flamingo pond, seemed somehow more at home than their more highly coloured, stilted companions.

More than for any other species, I felt sorry for the great cats. The lions and lionesses hadn't fared too badly at the hand of man. They had been allotted a rocky island surrounded by a deep moat, and despite the ever-present circle of pointing, camera-clicking people, they did have some semblance of limited freedom. Not so the tigers, cheetahs and jaguars. Confined to their cages, they would pace to and fro, with their great padded feet almost silent on the heavy boards. Their awesome power was occasionally seen when, as if to break the monotony, one would spring onto the top of its sleeping quarters in the corner of the cage and almost at once, leap down again to recommence its pacing routine. Perhaps the thing that concerned me most was the way they ignored their admiring public, who peered in on them from behind a restraining barrier a few feet from the cage front. The cats' eyes seemed to be fixed on something far beyond the visitors, the zoo, or even Edinburgh itself. I never once felt that these majestic animals had relinquished their desire for freedom and independence. Man may have captured and contained them, but he had most certainly not tamed them.

After all my early experiences of visiting and studying zoo animals at Edinburgh, it was not really surprising that I was somewhat attracted to becoming a zoo vet when I qualified from Glasgow Veterinary School. After all, I might be able to do something to improve the lot of captive animals. By this time I had also seen more of these exotic species on the many television wildlife programmes and had even had the occasional glimpse of the vets who specialized in this field. It certainly looked like a glamorous life to me! I managed to discount the occasion when one such zoo specialist, being filmed in an animal enclosure, was so intent on talking to the camera that he failed to evade a well-directed kick on his back end from a nearby giraffe!

As is often the case, glamorous goals had to take second place to the more practical business of earning a living and supporting a family. Some time later, however, I did have occasion to work with an exotic animal, and I too found out that it was not entirely without danger!

My first chance to work in front of a camera came when a freelance director asked if I could 'do a bit' in a film he was making.

A group called Compassion in World Farming had commissioned him to 'expose' the animal abuse that goes on in 'factory farming' where they believed that intensive methods of egg and meat production could lead to high levels of cruelty. The film was entitled 'Don't look now! Here comes your dinner'. This alone should have told me that it was not to be a wholly professional enterprise, but I was young and inexperienced and grabbed this opportunity to appear in a real film.

Before this momentous event in my life, I had done a great deal of public speaking and I had progressed through minor clubs and organizations to become quite adept at the job. So speaking was no big problem to me, but facing a camera was something else. Like most people I had the desire to 'perform' in public and to reap the rewards of others' applause. The only thing that was slightly holding me back was the fear of the consequences. What if I fail? What if the audience hates me? What if I die the death?

In my early days at Glasgow Veterinary School, I recall those same feelings. It happened when my fellow student and good friend Tom Begg asked me to be best man at his forthcoming wedding. Tom was a great chap, and in the closeness of our friendship, nobody would ever have suspected that he had gone to public school whereas I had attended the local comprehensive. Nor would anyone have imagined that his father was an eminent veterinary surgeon, whilst my dad had worked seven days a week in the coal mines to send me to university. Tom cared nothing about our different backgrounds, but to me they still mattered and I regretfully declined his invitation.

In my heart of hearts, I dearly wanted to be Tom's best man, for my sake as much as his, but the fear of failure made me chicken out. There would, I told myself, be lots of 'toffs' at the wedding, and as best man I would have to deliver a speech. The prospect of such a high-profile ordeal filled me with terror. In the months that followed, I never really forgave myself for my own inadequacy. Tom, after all, was my best friend and I had let him down.

A couple of years later I was offered the same 'honour' but this time by Jackie Oates, an old school friend of mine from Cowdenbeath. Jackie had left school to become a salesman, whereas I had stayed on, taken my Highers and eventually become a student at Glasgow University. Acceptance of Jackie's request had nothing to do with my apparently more elevated position in life. In fact it was quite the opposite. Jackie Oates and I were still, at heart, both working-class lads from the same mining town. We both knew each-other's families, relatives and friends. We were both from the same mould and I knew I would feel much more at home at his wedding with 'our kind of folk'.

Come Jackie and Wilma's big day, I stood up to give my first ever 'performance' in front of an audience. I would be lying if I said I wasn't nervous. It was, however, a natural kind of nervousness that comes from a pounding heart pumping adrenaline through your body in the expectancy of making an extra special effort. Then as now, I realized the all-important need to be well-prepared, but I also relied upon a 'talking technique' which I still use today.

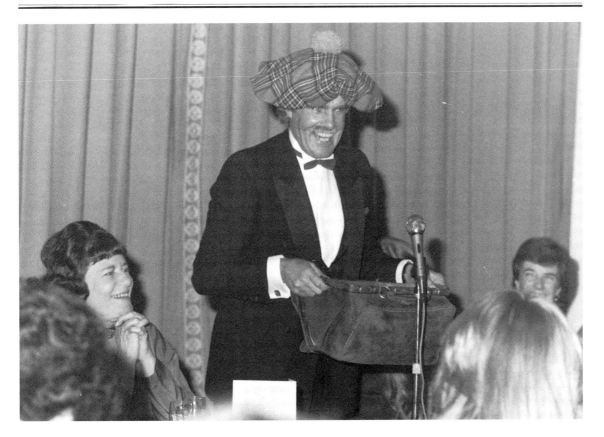

A tartan Tam o'Shanter and a musical medical bag help to add a little humour to an after-dinner performance.

I had watched other speakers, both at university and elsewhere, and when they used written notes it always seemed to limit their style somehow. So I elected to use only 'headlines' to guide me through my rehearsed speech and back up my act with a set of relevant props.

'Human beings,' my professor at college used to say, 'are visual animals, who are most impressed by what they see with their own eyes. The other senses of hearing, touch, smell and taste are important but they pale into insignificance when compared with the power of sight!'

From the moment I held up that brightly coloured plastic case, and turned it around to show the words printed upon it 'Best Man's Do-it-Yourself Kit' I had the audience eating out of my hand. From inside the case, I produced a giant hypodermic syringe fitted with a suitably long needle, and informed the audience that this was to revive the groom should he feel faint at the ceremony! On the ever-popular theme of the best man losing the ring, I confessed to the audience that I was not about to get caught out even if the worst happened. So saying I slowly pulled a dozen brass curtain rings linked together with thread from my top pocket! At the conclusion of my speech, I thanked all concerned but especially my own wife Alice.

'After all,' I said, tongue in cheek, 'it was she who kindly gave me some time off to perform my duties as best man.' As I said this I extended my right arm and a pair of policemen's handcuffs, attached to my wrist, dropped down to make my point!

Jackie and his new bride laughed heartily and the entire wedding party erupted into spontaneous applause. I loved it!

I was in the gents a little later, when two other wedding guests came in. Unaware of my presence, they gave me the best accolade of all.

'Did you hear that best man? asked one, 'Wasn't he bloody marvellous?'

'He sure was!' replied his companion enthusiastically and added, 'I only wish I could stand up and give a talk like that.'

Flushed with pride, I made a hurried exit.

In the ensuing years, I must have spoken to every conceivable kind of group and quickly discovered that no two talks or audiences are ever quite the same.

The 'upwardly mobile' middle-aged men of the Round Tables would always try to score points off the speaker but this only served to sharpen my skills in repartee. The women of the W.I., by contrast, just welcomed me for what I was and seemed delighted that I had taken the trouble to come along to tell them about my life as a vet. On one occasion, I was coming back into the hall to pick up my slide projector after a performance, when I was met head on by a lady who was just leaving.

'Thank you,' she said with genuine feeling, 'for being so wonderfully funny, but still managing to get across some serious messages.'

In gratitude for the compliment I kissed her on the cheek and wished her goodnight. Unfortunately all of the two hundred ladies who followed on behind her thought that the goodnight kiss was all part of my standard procedure! My departure may have been a little delayed that evening, but the ladies seemed to appreciate it!

One of the most dramatic incidents of my speaking career occurred when I was asked to give a talk to a club which attracts its members from the ranks of retired business and professional people. The chairman gave me a bit of a shock when he began by asking for the audience's attention and their sympathy while he read out the list of members who had 'passed away' since the last meeting! I made a mental note to increase the volume of my delivery and thanked my lucky stars that most of my material was visual!

About halfway through my slide talk, I heard a distinct grunt from about midway down the small hall, and thinking that it might mark someone's disapproval of my performance, I tried to focus my eyes on the source of the sound. In the dimly lit room, I could just make out the figure of an old man, slumped unnaturally in his seat. Had I not reached a particularly exciting part of my show, I might have suspected that the old gent had merely fallen asleep. There was, however, something about his posture that made me stop the talk and ask for the lights to be turned on. Amidst mumbled protests about this unscheduled interruption, I jumped from the stage and hurriedly made my way to the old man's seat.

His complexion was ashen. His body lay slumped at an awkward angle, and saliva drooled from the down-turned corner of his mouth. I also noticed, but didn't draw attention to the fact, that he had wet himself. As I felt his weak thready pulse I had already decided that the old man had had a stroke and asked the members gathered round me if there was a doctor in their midst. When the only doctor member was found, he appeared somewhat reluctant to offer any help. Indeed he seemed keener to impress upon me that he was long retired from active medical practice and very much out of touch. It soon became obvious that here was a very old doctor, in name only, who had long since lost the ability or the desire to make life and death decisions.

Ah well! Perhaps in this situation, a young vet might be able to offer more help than an ancient doctor, I decided, and sent him to phone for an ambulance.

As we waited, the patient suddenly regained consciousness. 'How do you feel?' I asked him.

A bit bewildered, he scanned the faces of the club members who were grouped around him. 'What's going on?' he asked as if the whole affair had nothing to do with him.

At that moment the doctor, flushed with his unexpected involvement in a medical emergency, returned to announce the imminent arrival of the ambulance. I considered it opportune to explain to my first human patient what I thought had happened.

'I think' I said quietly to him, 'you have had a little bit of a "funny turn".' I avoided using the word 'stroke' in case it might alarm him too much. 'But, never mind,' I assured him 'the ambulance will be here any minute, and we will get you off home.'

'Bugger that,' he said indignantly. 'The ambulance can wait. I want to see the rest of the show.'

I suppose that it was quite a compliment to me that we had to force him into the ambulance and I always wondered if he survived the experience or joined the list to be read out before the next meeting.

As a member of the veterinary profession, I naturally gave a lot of talks to groups of other vets. Sometimes, they were on serious subjects of medical or surgical interest, and at other times they were of the after-dinner variety. Among my props for the latter was an old-fashioned medical bag, which contained all the items that would lead me through my routine. Its most important feature, however, was a tape recorder built into the bottom of the bag. When I opened it, I could trigger a concealed micro switch and the bag would loudly play the 'Doctor Kildare' theme. Medical people like to poke fun at other medics and the musical bag proved to be a great prop for 'warming up' an audience.

Because of my work in a low temperature surgical technique called cryosurgery, I was invited to speak in Florida to the American College of Cryosurgery. For me, this was a very proud moment. I was a Scottish pet vet and now I had the honour of being asked to lecture to 'human' surgeons in the great US of A! Little did I realize however, that my real challenge was to come even before the plane touched down in Orlando.

Having settled down in one of the comfortable seats of the massive Tri-Star aircraft, I read through the inflight magazine, dismissed the temptation of the duty free, and eventually got into conversation with the young lady who sat next to me. She, it turned out, was a coronary care nurse, and when her husband learned that I was a vet, he didn't seem to mind, so much, that we were enthusiastically interested in each other's fields of medicine.

About a couple of hours into the journey, the head steward called for our attention over the tannoy. In a most respectful American accent he asked if there was 'a doctor of medicine' on the flight. I could soon see that there was not to be a volunteer, so I suggested to my new-found friend, that a nurse was the next best thing. Although she was a little reticent, I promised my moral support, and together we offered our 'expert' help. The head steward, now in a more hushed voice, confided in us that the medical problem was of a rather delicate nature.

'There is a young lady,' he told us, 'who has dislocated her ankle.' He hesitated, as the nurse and I looked in disbelief at each other. 'But,' said the steward leaning closer to us and lowering his voice even further, 'there is another complication. She is actually seated in one of the toilets!'

Anyone who has ever been in an aircraft will know that the toilets are scarcely big enough to turn around in and my mind struggled with the problem of how a young passenger had managed to dislocate her ankle in there in the first place! The steward, unconcerned with such medical trivia, hurried his two new-found allies to the scene of the young lady's dilemma.

On the way up the plane towards the toilet, the nurse was at great pains to explain to me that although she knew all about the blood supply to the heart, she understood very little about joint dislocations. I knew then that I was going to be in the driving seat, and when the toilet door was edged open, the nurse meaningfully pushed me to the front.

There, sitting on the toilet, was indeed a young lady, but her expression was not one of embarrassment, but of pain. The reason for this was obvious both to me and to the nurse. In fact, even someone with no medical knowledge at all would have been able to appreciate the problem. Her right foot was dislocated at the ankle joint and had twisted out of position so that it now lay at right angles to the rest of her leg.

Treating her just as I would a dog with a similar injury, I knelt down to examine the area as the nurse consoled the patient over my shoulder. I gently but firmly grasped the dislocated foot in my left hand, and took hold of the young lady's lower leg with my right hand to lock it in position. I looked up into her apprehensive eyes.

'I'm afraid that this is going to hurt a bit, darling,' I said. 'Are you all right?' She nodded and gave me a weak smile of encouragement.

I mentally crossed my fingers and using all my strength, snapped the dislocated foot back into alignment. It took quite an effort, but going by the smiles all around, the young lady's foot now looked as it should. Using the aircraft's medical kit, I put a retaining bandage on the ankle, after which we all retired from the toilet to allow the patient a little privacy to pull her pants up!

Now that the dramatic need for action was over, we helped the young lady to one of the crew seats, where we could get her leg up on a cushioned support. I then questioned a much more relaxed patient on how she had managed to dislocate her ankle. It transpired that she had been afflicted for some time with a ligament weakness which had made her joints unstable. Apparently she had suffered previous dislocations, but never before in such an awkward location!

At a stop-over in Bangor Maine airport the paramedics, summoned by the pilot, took our patient off for more specialized medical attention. Before leaving they took time to compliment the nurse and myself on the quality of our emergency treatment. The highlight of our performance was, however, when all the passengers on the aircraft burst into spontaneous applause in appreciation of our efforts.

Later, in a rare moment of relaxation at Disney World in Orlando, I bumped into the very same young lady. She had a plaster cast up to her knee, but was enjoying the rest of her holiday, being pushed around in a wheelchair. She didn't seem at all embarrassed by her bathroom experience at thirty-seven thousand feet!

I had a great time at the cryosurgery conference in America and perhaps the only black spot was created by a rather stuffy Harley Street consultant. He tried to 'do down' the American audience in his opening remarks.

'Although the declared language of this conference has been designated to be English,' he commenced with very precise diction, 'in my estimation, my paper will be the first to be truly delivered in that language!' This snobbish attitude not only threatened to switch off the audience, but could have made it difficult for me to follow him, as I was next on. Fortunately, I have always enjoyed ad-libbing, so it was no problem to change round the previously planned opening for my paper.

'Ladies and Gentlemen, this afternoon my contribution will not,' I stressed, 'be delivered in English.' The audience warmed to me. 'In a very few moments,' I went on, accentuating my Scottish accent, 'you are going to realize that neither am I an American!' This light relief won the day, and when my first slide showed me wearing full Scottish Highland dress, I had them all on my side.

'Lower your eyes,' I told them, tongue in cheek, 'if you are of a nervous disposition. Because,' I hesitated, scanning a medical audience who were quite accustomed to seeing everything from piles to brain tumours, 'I am about to show you something which you may find shocking.' Before they could even start to guess at what this might be, I continued.

'Everyone in the world,' I said emphatically, 'wants to know what a Scotsman wears under his kilt.' The audience went deadly quiet in anticipation.

My finger poised on the button of the slide changer, I glanced over my shoulder at the full-length picture of myself in Highland attire. I hit the button. The slide changed. There I was, hoisting my kilt high enough to show my underpants, but with the most important portion delicately covered by a mini tartan hot water bottle. On it were the simple words, 'Willie warmer'. The audience fell about laughing. I was on my way, and the spectre of the Harley Street bum had been laid to rest.

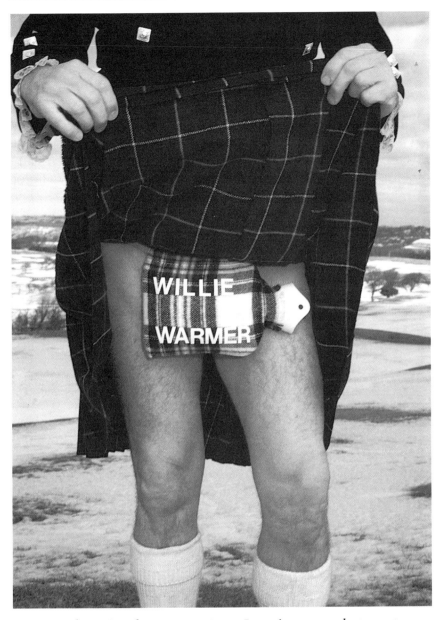

Most people want to know what a Scotsman wears under his kilt. I was courageous enough to reveal all to an American audience.

Of all the talks I have ever given, I am fortunate that most were enthusiastically received. By my own reckoning, I have only 'plumbed the depths' on one occasion. This was relatively recently when, as an established TV personality, I was persuaded to perform as an after-dinner speaker for the Captain's Night at a well-known golf club.

I arrived at seven o'clock with the captain and after a long evening of in-jokes and revelry, I stood up to do my bit at around half past midnight. As a professional, I was stone-cold sober, which was more than I can say for my audience. To a man, they were sozzled. Knocking back wine and spirits, as if to proclaim their affluence to each other, they pulled on big cigars and, through a drunken haze, reluctantly sneered a welcome to this outsider. Although I did my professional best that night, I scored myself pretty poorly and swore never to speak to another collection of such non-sporting sportsmen. However, in the cold light of the next morning, I was forced to admit that the audience is never wrong and that my mistake was accepting the engagement in the first place. I just didn't fit into that scene and that troubled me not at all!

By contrast, I was once called upon to fill in for the Under Secretary of State at very short notice. That, I reckoned, had to be some sort of first for a miner's son from Cowdenbeath! Apparently, this eminent politician was under a three-line whip at the House of Commons and could not meet his speaking engagement. His intended audience, the chiefs of all the Electricity Boards in the country and many of their influential friends, were assembled at the Majestic Hotel in Harrogate.

'Is there any chance, John,' asked a distraught controller of leisure activities, 'that you could fill in for him?'

It was now lunchtime and I would have to perform at seven-thirty that evening. I was apprehensive. I was scared. No, let's face it, I was terrified!

'Of course,' I said, as confidently as I could. 'Tell me about the audience and the fee.'

That night, with a red-coated toastmaster in attendance, I sat next to Sir So and So and when the time came for my speech, I hit them with everything I had. I started with a light-hearted joke about electricity, but from then on in, it was down to the musical medical bag and tales of my life as a vet. They loved it, and did not seem to mind that my speech had nothing to do with politics.

Of all the many talks I have given to groups as far removed as Florida surgeons, English fish-egg importers and Finnish plywood manufacturers, the most memorable of all must be the one I gave to the NATN: The National Association of Theatre Nurses.

This group of wonderful and dedicated ladies meets annually in Harrogate and after attending a programme of serious lectures, they let their hair down at their annual dinner on the Saturday evening. The first after-dinner speaker was a well-known expert on the human urinary system, a urologist, and I was to follow him. From the moment I stood up and announced that I was a vet, I had their sympathetic approval. When I joked that I had always thought that urologists mended clocks, the nurses took me to their hearts. They loved my musical bag and all the medical props it contained.

At the end of my talk, they all rose to their feet and gave me a standing ovation. I can tell you that was quite something! Most of us have reason to be grateful to nurses at some time or other, but to have five hundred of them on their feet applauding my performance, must truly have been the highlight of my speaking career.

After a suitable space of time, where so many of my audience approached and thanked me personally, I headed upstairs to my hotel room, where my wife Alice waited for me. I never liked her to come to my talks, perhaps again because of my working-class fear of failure.

As I fairly bounded into the room, my breast full of righteous pride, I blurted out, 'Alice...you'll never guess...'

I never actually got out the bit about the standing ovation, because Alice, turning from the television, put her finger to her lips and said loudly, 'Sh! Sh! I'm just watching the end of this programme!'

It was then, at that very moment, that I realized two things: what is important to us may not be so important to others, and also that the power of television is great indeed!

Now, with this rich mixture of public speaking experience under my belt, I was about to make my first film and I knew absolutely nothing about appearing in front of a camera. It did not take me long, however, to discover what a low-budget film shoot was all about!

In order to make a little profit for himself, the director had to cut corners. Being a Glaswegian with more than a little charm and persuasiveness built in to his personality, his first trick was to hire the entire cast for nothing! The film crew, already hardened in the television industry, came slightly more expensive.

First day out, my young mind found reward enough in learning how a film is actually made, and despite the lack of money and an entirely amateur cast, I enjoyed every minute of it. As it was an animal-based film it was not surprising that I, as a vet, had the starring role. When I said something about animals my professional status would give it authority. This fact may have been the director's real reason for casting me, and this didn't help increase my self-confidence. It was some compensation to know that none of the other performers were any more professional at acting than I was.

The theme of the film was a dream sequence where the son of the director's next-door neighbour is taken from the arms of his loving mother, played incidentally by his loving mother, and subjected to

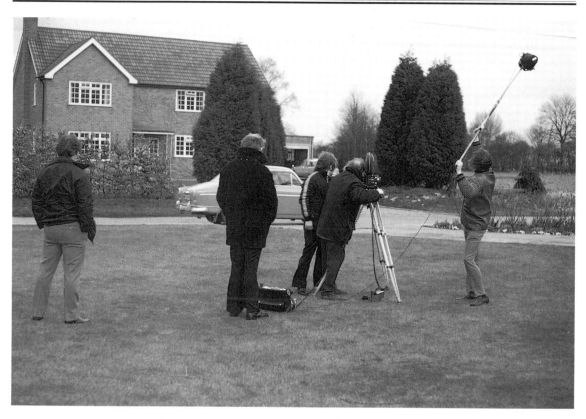

The crew gets ready to film a scene in 'Don't Look Now – Here Comes Your Dinner!'. Admittedly, it is a terrible title, but it was my first time on film.

the treatment that a young pig has to endure before being slaughtered for food. The idea was to invite the audience to put themselves in the position of animals, down on the farm that have to experience such horrors.

In another sequence, the director wanted to show how modern living has influenced our relationship with animals. High-rise flat accommodation and high-speed motorways have a damaging effect. One part of the film showed a crow and a very obviously stuffed crow at that, standing by the motorway, watching as the vehicles roared past. Next, the director cut to the green fields and then swung the camera back to the motorway, where the stuffed crow was now lying 'dead' on its side. Obviously a victim of modern living! Even in my state of inexperience I would have edited that part out of the film.

Perhaps my most lasting memory of that first film was when the director asked me to lean casually on a calf and start pontificating about beef production in Great Britain. The fact that I was a pet vet and knew virtually nothing about farm animals was neither here nor there. What seemed really important to the crew was keeping the calf still, while I delivered my lines. Then in true film style, I was to pat the calf affectionately on its rump and walk nonchalantly towards the door of a nearby shed.

'Cut!' shouted the director, in true Hollywood style. 'Okay. Reset for the reverse.'

All of this jargon sounded good, but quite meaningless, to me, until he explained that the crew would now set up the camera, with mikes and lights inside the cattle shed, and when I opened the door and walked in, it would look realistic.

As I stood alone, outside that door, dressed head to toe in blue denim, I stroked my Jason King moustache and awaited the next part of my performance with some anxiety.

From inside, I heard the director's call for 'Action!' I counted to ten and opened the door. Facing me was a long concrete corridor bordered by three-foot walls which enclosed pens on either side, where young beef cattle were housed. From that day to this, I still find that the hardest part of film work is walking 'naturally' towards the position where I will turn and talk to the camera. Picking up a couple of concentrated food pellets from the troughs which lay at intervals along the wall, I walked down the corridor to reach my pre-marked spot. As I glanced at the cattle on either side, in an attempt to look relaxed, I tried hard not to beam in on the chalk mark which lay ahead, nor to look directly at the camera. By the time I reached the mark, my heart was pounding and I was rolling the food pellets in my fingers as if, somehow, their agitation would lessen mine. I leaned casually against the wall with my elbow resting on its top and began my piece to camera.

'The British farmer,' I said, hoping my Scottish accent and my fashionable denim jacket would somehow conceal the tremor in my voice, 'is among the top exponents of animal husbandry in the whole world...'

As I droned on with my words of wisdom, I was completely oblivious to everything around me. The cattle, being inquisitive animals, were not! One beast, whose curiosity combined well with a bold personality, was so intrigued by this denim-clad apparition, that it came right up to my side and started to lick enthusiastically at my elbow. I was so intent on my delivery that I never even noticed. The camera, that all-seeing eye, caught every detail!

As the cow licked, the blue colour of the denim deepened and like a piece of blotting paper, the process continued up my arm, as the cow's saliva soaked relentlessly up to my shoulder. My heart still thumping, I finished my spiel and only then questioned how my sleeve had so suddenly become sodden!

That film was not only paid for by Compassion in World Farming, but went on to convince its devotees that the cause they all fought for was a worthy one. Despite my sometimes laughable performances, and my coat of many colours, I was quite a short-lived hero in their ranks. As the 'star' I was even invited to a showing of the film in London and when the lights went up at its end, there wasn't a dry eye in the house. Nobody seemed to have even noticed my nerves or my deep-blue sleeve!

I still have the large round can which contains the original sixteen-millimetre film, and although my current TV crew fall about laughing at its format and contents, for me it still holds a unique position in my film career.

Chapter 2

Vet on Screen

My television career began when a local TV producer rang me up and asked if I could 'do a little animal spot', as he put it, 'with a selection of furry creatures and their owners'.

Now if there is one animal you have got to be wary of and watch more closely than any pet or zoo animal, it is that rare species called a television producer! I should have known that fellow Scot, Graham Ironside, would have a little surprise in store for me. Designed, no doubt, to liven up an already 'live' programme.

I arrived at the studio in good time, all dolled up in a swish new jacket that I had been saving for just such a special occasion. I looked good, I felt good, and I was more than ready for any quiet wee chat about children's pets.

I should have twigged that all was not well when the seasoned reporter welcomed me with obvious apprehension in his manner and took great pains to place me between himself and a little group of youngsters with their assorted pets. His sly glance in the direction of the children was enough to show me the cause of his concern. One little lad stood slightly apart from the others holding a brown canvas sack – and the sack was moving! There was no time now for me to worry about its contents, but after dispensing with rabbits, hamsters, mice and guinea pigs, I couldn't just leave him standing there – holding that moving bag! It didn't help when the television interviewer cued me in by taking two steps back. The three big studio cameras beamed in as if to show the world what kind of man I really was.

I swallowed hard and asked the simple question, 'Well now son, what have you got in your bag?' I tried to sound confident – but the beating of my heart was a more honest reflection of my feelings.

'It's a royal python,' the boy replied enthusiastically, his eyes shining with the certain knowledge that being a vet I couldn't fail to know all about snakes and love them wholeheartedly.

How was he to know that my experience of snakes was limited to say the least. All I knew was that some were venomous and could poison you with one bite from their hollow fangs, whilst others were constrictor snakes that had relinquished the venom weapon in favour of crushing their victims to death in their muscular coils! The only other relatively useless fact I knew about snakes was that they could totally empty their bowels if they got frightened. This pittance of knowledge sped through my mind in milliseconds.

'Is he dangerous?' I asked, putting on a rather overdone smile.

'Well,' said the lad, obviously blissfully unaware of my fear, 'he did bite my brother.' As the smile slid from my face, he added 'But he was afraid of it!'

I quickly switched on a rather watery expression in an ineffectual attempt to conceal that I too was not exactly brimming over with confidence.

Such is the power of television, however, that for some inexplicable reason I heard myself asking to see the creature!

After that, everything apart from the giant eight-feet-long royal python, was 'out of my hands'. Before I had time to bat an eyelid or beat a respectful retreat, the reptile had slithered regally out of the neck of the sack and was coursing its way through my outstretched hands, over my arms and commencing its first coil round my body. As more and more of the snake slid from the sack, I could feel its rippling muscular power as it wound itself around me.

Nervously, I faced the camera and explained that pythons were not venomous snakes that killed their prey with poisonous bites. No! They were constrictor snakes that crushed their victims to death by restricting their ability to breathe! This particular python made the point by taking another turn around my trembling frame.

'You know,' I said, feeling that I must impart some knowledge to warrant the risks I was running, 'snakes are not really pets, they are more of a specialized hobby.' And, I thought to myself, as coil three entwined my body, there is a tendency for all snakes to defecate if they get too excited. Here I was standing in my very best expensive jacket – bought specially for the occasion – with eight feet of royal python wrapped round me, amidst the lights, cameras and all the other technical paraphernalia of television.

All my fears for my jacket and appearance were short-lived as I felt the python's head hovering around my left ear. The little lad's words resounded like some prophecy of doom in my brain. 'Well, he did bite my brother.'

'And so,' I said in conclusion, thankful not to have a tattered ear, a ruined jacket and a dented reputation, 'snakes are best left to the specialist.' I must admit that I half hoped that any snake fanciers out there in the viewing public would know that I certainly did not come into this category!

As the closing music played and the royal python finished his winding course majestically poised over the top of my head, I had to admit that it did look spectacular on the monitor.

The young lad helped unwind me from his beloved snake and the television crew complimented me – still from a safe distance, and I took a deep breath and felt good. After all, my jacket was still in pristine condition and what is more important, so was my ear.

'What did you think, Alice?' I asked my wife, when I burst enthusiastically back into my home after the programme. 'How did I do?' I demanded, my eyes sparkling in expectation of an accolade.

Alice looked up at me and with kindness tempering her reply said, 'Well it was all right – but let me put it this way – you looked absolutely terrified!'

Ah well, as Scotland's national poet once wrote in his wisdom 'O wad some Power the giftie gie us, to see oursels as ithers see us!'

Very true, and I had learned one of the important rules of being on television. The cameras and the viewing public can pick up almost every detail of your innermost soul, and even a swish new jacket can be a very poor cover-up!

Next morning I awoke with an air of expectancy. After all, I had made my first appearance on British television and despite that giant python, lived to tell the tale!

For my wife and family it was just another day, but for me, it was full of promise. My foot was firmly on the ladder of success and I was sure that any minute my friends would be on the phone pouring out their congratulations on my previous night's performance.

No such luck! The event passed as if it had never happened. Lasting success, I learned, is not built on one brief appearance on a television screen. I would have to work a good deal harder, if ever I was to become a 'star'.

The one thing that the snake episode did achieve, was to imprint me forever in the minds of the television reporters and other staff associated with that programme. Nothing sells you more effectively to television people than the ability to keep speaking whilst in a life-threatening situation. Creating an interesting spectacle is their business and if you can make this as dramatic as possible then you are 'in'!

Over the next months, I did lots of little spots on the local

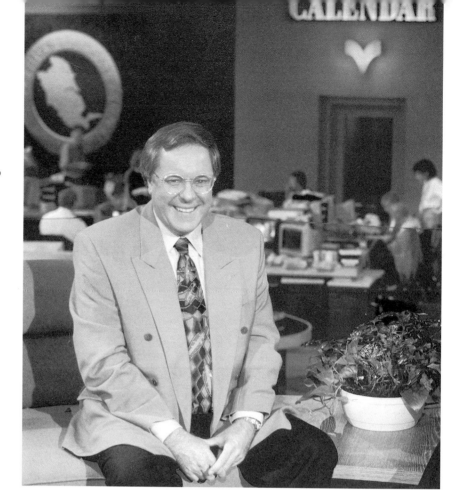

Richard Whiteley, presenter of Yorkshire Television's 'Calendar' news programme, and the popular Channel Four quiz show 'Countdown', helped to launch me on to television.

'Calendar' news programme and although nothing ever quite matched the python, I did manage to impress several producers with my television presence. In my capacity as a vet, I even appeared as Father Christmas with a live reindeer.

Then came my big break. The head of local programmes, Graham Ironside rang me to do what I thought was another spot on Yorkshire Television's 'Calendar'.

'Do you think, John,' he asked persuasively, 'you could do half-an-hour live?' My momentary hesitation was only because I wasn't quite sure what half-an-hour live meant.

'Of course, Graham,' I replied, trying to sound more confident than I really was, 'I'd love to, but what is it all about?'

'Well John,' he said, now warming to the prospect, 'you know we run a programme which goes out at three-thirty in the afternoon called 'Calendar Tuesday'. Have you ever caught it?'

In truth, being a busy practising vet, my afternoons were more likely to be taken up with broken bones or bleeding patients than watching television, but somehow the absolute truth seemed inappropriate at that moment.

'Aye, I have, Graham. I have seen it on the odd occasion.' I lied, but continued, 'It's a good programme.'

'Aye, okay John,' replied Graham, relaxing into his 'fellow Scot' accent. 'Then you will know that the format is for Richard Whiteley to interview a celebrity.' He hesitated, then went on: 'Well the intended celebrity cannae make it and we wondered if you would like to have a go?'

Now if there was one thing I wasn't, it was a celebrity. This, however, was too good a chance to miss. I wanted to do a bit of television, I knew that I could talk, so this could be a heaven-sent opportunity.

'Great!' said Graham, in response to my acceptance. 'We'll see you at the studios about two o'clock on Tuesday. That will give you a chance to have a chat with Richard before the show. Oh, and by the way, John,' he added, 'we will have a few wee animals for you to refer to.'

Graham was off the phone and away before I could ask him if there was a python among them. I sat down both breathless and excited, but most definitely looking forward to the following Tuesday.

On Monday, I spent a fitful night worrying about the 'live' performance to come the following afternoon. I had done all I could to make as good a visual impression as possible. New grey trousers, a smart navy jacket and a crisp new white shirt with a very professional-looking tie. My hair, having been cut three days previously, now looked naturally well-groomed. The rest, I decided, was up to my brain, my mouth and a modicum of good luck.

I had reckoned without several factors, one of which was Richard Whiteley.

I arrived early at the studios of Yorkshire Television and sheepishly informed the security man that I was there to do 'Calendar Tuesday'. Despite my many appearances on the News programmes, he didn't know me from Adam! His doubt about this 'unknown celebrity' was soon cancelled by a quick phone call and I was allowed to pass through the foyer to the inner sanctum.

I had arranged to meet the programme production assistant in the canteen, but being early, I had time to drink two cups of coffee before the agreed time. Looking furtively around the room, and trying not to look too new, I spotted a couple of real personalities mingling with television staff. They were trying to look ordinary and this only made me feel more of a phoney.

'So here you are, John.' I nearly choked on the remains of my second cup as the PA plonked her hand on my shoulder. 'Everything all right?' she asked, giving me a beaming smile of reassurance. This, I realized later, was all part of her television stock in trade. PAs are wonderfully skilled people who are highly paid to know everything, cater for all the crew, and hold the programme together at all costs! 'If you have finished your coffee,' she continued, encouraging me by moving her hand to my elbow to help me up, 'I'll get you through to make-up.'

'I'll have to make a short stop at the toilets,' I retorted, as I felt the effects of the coffee on my kidneys.

'No problem. It's on the way,' she said, rekindling her smile and striding out of the canteen.

However, disaster struck as I turned on the tap to wash my hands. The jet of water hit the porcelain with such force that it shot round the bowl, came over the side and soaked my previously immaculate grey flannels! What was I to do? No one would ever believe I hadn't wet myself in quite another way. To cap it all, the PA was bound to be getting restless outside the toilet door.

'I'll only be a couple of minutes,' I shouted, as I unfastened my trousers and hung them over the hot air hand dryer. Red-faced with the heat and the effort, I emerged to meet the puzzled expression of the PA and decided there and then that grey trousers were 'out' for television appearances.

In make-up, a charming and pretty young lady settled me back in the chair and delicately fastened a cover-all around my neck.

'Well,' she said reassuringly, talking to my image in the mirror, 'I haven't got much to do for you.' She proceeded to dust a little powder on my rather flushed face and drew a soothing comb through my hair. Taking off the cover-all with a cheery 'There you go then. You look wonderful!' she pronounced me ready for my performance and did wonders for my ego.

Just as I was beginning to feel good, the PA returned and whisked me off to meet Richard Whiteley. He was already seated on the interviewing couch and around him were several pet animals and on a table in front, a goldfish bowl. I was pleased to note that there were no sacks or other receptacles which might have contained a snake.

Richard, if anything, looked slightly more nervous than I felt. He was obviously intent on setting things up and only glanced in my general direction to acknowledge my arrival. Not quite the friendly encouragement I had expected from a man of his many years of television experience. Then again, he perhaps felt that dealing with a non-celebrity might make for added problems.

Eventually he finished his conversation via microphone and

earpiece with the director who was hidden somewhere high above us, and turned at last to put me at my ease.

'Now John,' he started, 'we'll just be having a bit of a chat about you and your life as a vet and maybe use some of these animals as background material.'

I pointed at the goldfish bowl. 'Don't ask me about fish,' I advised, 'because I know very little about them, but anything else is okay.'

Of course, I now realize that that is the last thing you want to tell a reporter. When the titles rolled, and the show got under way, you can guess the first question he asked me.

'Now then John, these goldfish look pretty bored. Why do you think that is?'

Quick as a flash, I replied, 'Well Richard, I think that's anthropomorphism,' and then hesitated for his response.

Whether he thought that this was some new psychological disease of goldfish which made them looked bored, I do not know, but if his expression was anything to go by, he certainly didn't comprehend that anthropomorphism means attributing human feelings to animals. If anything, he looked even more vacant than the fish. The cameraman was quick to tighten on a head shot and as the director held the close-up of Richard's face, the entire viewing public knew he didn't understand, as he moved on to his next question.

For me, the whole programme then became great fun, and to be fair to Richard, he not only brought out the best in me, but really seemed to enjoy himself.

As soon as the programme was over, Graham was down on the studio floor, complimenting Richard and myself on the quality of the show. Later that day, I headed home a happier and wiser man.

Unknown to me, Graham and myself were not the only people who were impressed by my performance. Forced to stay at home by a bad bout of flu, a prominent TV producer called John Meade had caught the programme.

No sooner had I got back home than the telephone rang and, amidst coughs and sneezes, John Meade introduced himself and said he would like to meet me to discuss a possible series.

In the years to come, I was to learn so much about making programmes from this talented and innovative producer, but for now I was just flattered to be wanted on the box.

I had thoroughly enjoyed being a guest on 'Calendar Tuesday', and loved being a 'substitute star': if that was television, I wanted more of it.

Chapter 3

Starring Role

'Everything all right, darlings?' The smiling floor manager leaned forward, then, just as swiftly, backed off again, answering his own question.

'Okay. Thirty seconds to camera!'

I glanced anxiously to my left, where my colleague, Marylyn, was making a final check on her opening lines. Over to my right, a group of my clients sat nervously, over-fondling their pets.

This was it! The very first programme of my very own television series, and here I was, standing in a real television studio. I was terrified!

I cracked some inane pleasantry to Marylyn, who should have been used to this sort of thing, but appeared just as apprehensive as I was. I took a deep breath and looked out onto the studio floor ahead of me.

What was it the director had told me? The camera on the left was mine, but that was called 'camera right' in television jargon. The one on the right was Marylyn's and the one straight ahead would take the wide shots. Or was it the other way round?

Before my befuddled brain could sort things out, the floor manager, complete with headphones and walkie-talkie, was back. This time, he came much closer to us, his manner now tinged with urgency.

'Ten seconds to camera,' he said, this time without a smile, and held up both hands with the fingers extended, in case we had gone deaf with fright.

The ten seconds passed in a flash and almost before I knew it the strident clarion call of Yorkshire Television's standard musical introduction shocked me back into conscious awareness of my situation.

'Tah Tah Rah Tah Tah!' it blared out across the studio. Had it been announcing the triumphant arrival of Genghis Khan and his hordes into Studio Two, it could not have made more impact on me. No wonder the 'professionals' called it the 'Sting'.

The three huge studio cameras glided towards us, like great devocalized Daleks and zoomed in as if to pick up my every faltering word and expression.

We were on! This was the big time! The miracle is that I did not fall into a dead faint on the spot.

'Hello and welcome to the very first programme of a brand new series called "It's a Vet's Life"' Marylyn announced in her best professional newscaster's voice. She had been on the local 'Calendar' news team for several years, so was well used to working in front of the camera. 'This is a series,' she continued, 'about animals with problems and about the vets who do their best to get them back to health, and,' she went on, 'the vet next to me, is my co-presenter, John Baxter.'

Turning from her auto-cue, which helped explain her word-perfect start, Marylyn launched me into the world of television, with her first question. 'Now John, what are you going to tell us about today?'

Standing there in a mocked-up studio set, built to look like my own surgery, I picked up a three-foot-long prop bone from the table and immediately realized two very important things. The first was that television is a visual medium and viewers need to see interesting things on the screen. The second was that I felt completely in my element. Nervous or not, I liked being on TV!

In the ensuing discussion on the medical folly of giving a dog a bone, I used a multitude of other props, such as x-rays and real bone fragments to make my points. Then the floor manager with a circular motion of his arm, indicated that I should 'wind up this piece', and then, with a final stroke of his flattened hand across his throat, instructed me to 'cut'.

With the first segment completed, there now followed a three-minute piece of film which had been previously shot on location. This gave me time to get my act together. What a blessed relief that was! As the film section was being electronically edited onto our opening, I looked across at my guests and their pets, who had been assembled to make up a TV version of a clinic.

This bit should go well, I thought. After all, I had had a 'run-through' with them before the recording and I knew, pretty well, what we should all be doing.

At the head of the queue sat Mrs Dobson with her duck George, confined to a cat basket. In the run-through, Mrs Dobson's nerves and a faulty catch on the cage door, had conspired to make George's appearance a much-delayed event. In television, I was soon to learn, everything has to be short and snappy, so we finally elected to keep the cage door closed, but unlatched. Next to Mrs Dobson sat Mrs Wilson with her dog. Mrs Wilson was, to say the least, a very large lady. She once boasted to me in my real consulting room, that she could lose three stones' body weight in no time at all. When I had looked slightly sceptical, a jovial Mrs Wilson explained that all she would have to do would be 'to have a leg removed'.

Mrs Wilson did everything in a 'big' way and her choice of dogs was no different. Fortunately the massive Newfoundland at the other end of her lead was as placid and manageable as Mrs Wilson wasn't!

At the back of the queue, separated from Mrs Wilson by a Green Iguana with a diet problem, a rabbit with a slipped disc and an itchy guinea pig, sat Mr Roberts with his Rottweiler. This separation was the floor manager's most effective piece of floor managing. In the rehearsal before the recording began, the two dogs had not been so far apart and the Rottie had decided to have a go at the big Newfoundland. In the normal run of things, the Rottie would have won hands down, but he reckoned without Mrs Wilson. Years of running a pub in one of the rougher areas of the city had equipped her with a vast repertoire of expletives and the ability to tackle and evict the toughest of troublemakers. For Mrs Wilson, a Rottweiler was easy meat. As her great Newfoundland hid behind her bulk, she swung a well-directed three-stone kick at the Rottie's rear end, and the fracas was immediately over. Well, it would have been, except that in the fray, Mrs Wilson managed to ladder one leg of her tights.

In television, the wardrobe department is equipped and ready for all such eventualities and one of their staff was summoned to help. A well-rounded, hand-on-hip wardrobe man minced into the studio to sort things out.

'Now then' he said, touching his lips to heighten the drama, 'How can we help?'

If King Henry VIII had lost part of his codpiece, they could cope. If a presenter needed his suit pressed, or a ballet dancer tore her tutu, the wardrobe department could deliver. However, Mrs Wilson's tights proved to be their Waterloo! Nowhere in their vast stocks of clothing for all occasions was there a pair of tights big enough to fit her but never let it be said that television people are not resourceful. A motor cyclist was dispatched to Mrs Wilson's pub and with no help at all from the wardrobe man, Mrs Wilson was soon pulling herself into a second pair of voluminous tights. Now, she felt well-dressed enough to appear on the telly!

The floor manager, standing next to 'my camera', counted me out of the film with the fingers of his left hand next to the camera lens. He reinforced the countdown by silently mouthing 'Five, four, three, two,' and when he reached 'one', he stabbed his index finger directly at me, to indicate that I was 'on'!

I read the first few lines on the auto-cue, which rolled in large print, just under the camera lens and decided at that moment, it wasn't quite me. Ad-libbing was much more my style, and in any case, the animals and guests were ready and waiting, so I called over Mrs Dobson with her duck.

George was no ordinary duck. He was a kleptomaniac! For those of you who are unfamiliar with kleptomania, let me explain that it usually applies to humans who cannot resist stealing absolutely anything. In the animal world, magpies and jackdaws have earned something of a reputation for such behaviour, but George was the first kleptomaniac duck I had come across.

George was no ordinary duck – he was a duck with a desire to possess anything shiny that caught his eye: he was a kleptomaniac.

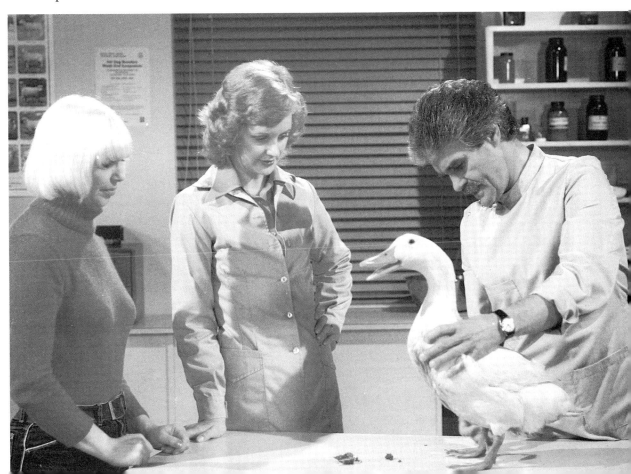

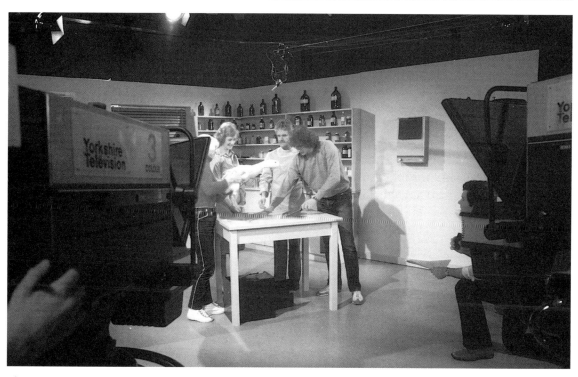

The studio cleaner had to be called in when George got over excited and blotted his copy book – in front of several million viewers.

Prior to this television appearance, I had taken George onto a local radio show as part of a programme featuring myself and some of my avian patients. I had a pigeon with a broken wing, an egg-bound budgie, a bald parrot and finally George, who was to be the star of the show. Because of the size of the performing cast, the reporter decided to do the interview, not at a table, but with the various birds and their owners standing round in a semi-circle in the radio studio. The plan was for the reporter to use a hand-held microphone and then he and I would pass from one case to the next, discussing each in turn. It all worked well until we came to George. As the reporter extended the microphone to get Mrs Dobson's comments on her duck's unusual condition, George spotted the shiny metallic rim on the front of the mike. 'That,' he decided, 'I have to have for my collection.' The reporter who, until that moment, had been most correct and very professional, thought that the duck was launching an attack on him, and momentarily lost his cool. As he leaped backwards, taking his mike with him, George took off from his owner's arms in hot pursuit. This only served to reinforce the reporter's belief that his life was in danger, and it took my veterinary intervention to grab George, conclude the interview and save the day. The sound quality of that session, doubtless to say, left a lot to be desired.

Whether it was that experience or just being on telly that affected Mrs Dobson, I will never know, but as she approached the table at my bidding, she was distinctly jittery.

'Just pop the cage on the table, Mrs Dobson,' I said, smiling to relieve her tension.

As she did so, disaster struck for a second time. In her state of nerves, Mrs Dobson's judgement was a bit out, and as she moved to place the cage on the table, the bottom of it caught the table edge. The impact caused the unlatched door to fly open, and a very surprised George shot into the full view of the studio cameras. That entrance would have been spectacular enough for most 'stars', but birds, like humans, do tend to be stimulated into certain actions by fear or shock. As George catapulted from the cage and came to rest 'centre stage', his excitement was such that he did 'you-know-what' right in the middle of the table.

W C Fields once said that you should never work with children or animals. I was beginning to think that he might have had a point!

Of course, television technology came to the rescue. George and the table were cleaned up and the piece repeated and then joined back on again with the magic of an 'add-on edit'. It would now look to the viewer as if George and Mrs Dobson had both given faultless performances, but I personally thought it made better television first time round!

Chapter 4

Camera Consultations

'Sit there like a good girl,' said Bernie, my nurse, as she plumped Pudding down on her rear end on the consulting-room table.

'Ian, just put a bit more scrim on that back light for me,' demanded Charlie, eager to tune up on the final niceties of getting the scene lit properly.

Ian, who combined his talents as both sound man and sparks, hoisted his slim six-foot frame onto a stool behind us and clipped some more white tissue over the eight-hundred-watt 'red head' to diffuse the light further. Pudding didn't move a muscle.

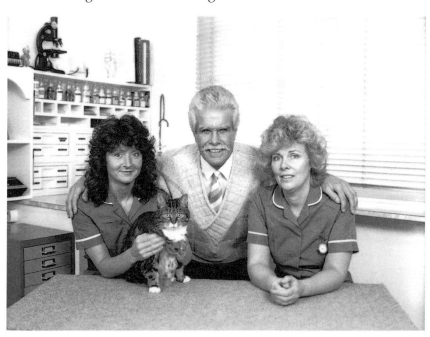

I am known by my staff at the surgery as Mr B, so I suppose it is natural enough for me to call them the B team.

'How's that, Charlie?' Ian asked, keen to avoid leaping down and then having to leap back up again.

Charlie took a look through the camera lens. 'Looks fine to me, Ian,' he said and, turning, asked 'How does it look on the monitor, Mike?'

Because of the smallness of my consulting room, now doubling as a studio, Mike Best the producer was seated round the corner on the stairs with a television monitor just in front of him. He poked his head round the corner, gave Charlie a thumbs-up sign, and nodded his approval.

'Fine,' he confirmed. Mike, despite his high degree of technical skill, was a man of few words.

I had learned over the years that if things were all right for Charlie, Mike and Ian, then they would surefire be okay by me!

Ian climbed down and resumed his position next to the camera, slipping on his headphones. Holding the 'cans' steady with one hand, he gave the knobs of his recording machine a final twiddle with the other, and then signalled his readiness to Charlie.

'Action!' said Charlie.

By this stage any ordinary cat would have been well gone but Pudding, perhaps one of the most filmed cats on British television, was a true professional and merely sat waiting for her cue. The general subject for this piece of filming was the pros and cons of being fat. Pudding's qualification for starring in this section was self-evident! Weighing in at thirteen pounds, she looked more like a stuffed pyjama case than a moggy. She was very much overweight.

'Hold her steady, Bernie, whilst I slip this measuring tape round her middle.' Pudding, who would do anything if there was the slightest prospect of food at the end of it, sat patiently as I threaded the yellow tape round her. As Bernie and I gasped in amazement at her girth, Pudding gave a kind of sigh. As a 'media' cat, she had heard it all before and she knew that if she performed well, someone or other would reward her with a bit extra in her food bowl!

There were several angles that the story could take. There were the problems which obesity could cause the heart, liver and lungs and, of course, the joints of the limbs which had to carry this excess bulk around. Also there were the added risks if surgery ever had to be performed on a fat animal and finally, the all too obvious fact that such an obese cat as Pudding belonged to a TV vet who had tried and failed to slim her down!

Pudding, or Fat Cat as we sometimes call her, had been adopted by the practice when her original owner had left town. She had been overweight then, and as her owner was out all day, she had learned to combine a joyful reunion with an ample dish of food. Since she had been nibbling away all day as well, it is not surprising that her body weight just went up and up! Now, Pudding expected any human contact to be accompanied by food, whether she was hungry or not. Love and affection were intimately linked to eating. If food was not forthcoming as we tried to break this bond, Pudding would use every alluring female wile she could to lead us towards the food bowl. When she felt that we were close enough, she would fall into a provocative pose on one side and stretch out a front paw. For all the world it looked as if she was pointing to her dish in a final attempt to make some dumb human 'get the message'.

Nevertheless, the staff and I set out scientifically to reduce her body weight by putting her on a strict calorie-controlled diet. Her food was weighed accurately and to the manufacturer's specification and we adhered rigidly to this for all of three months. When we weighed her, she had only lost half an ounce! The company couldn't believe it, but I could, because cats are totally different animals to dogs or even humans. If you don't give a cat sufficient calories, it will make up for its reduced intake by expending less energy. Pudding simply slept more.

'If you don't feed me,' she seemed to say, 'then I'm not going to walk around.'

We tried forcing her to exercise through play by throwing toy balls to her in the hope that she would run to retrieve them. Not Pudding! At most, she moved her eyes to watch the object as it passed in front of her line of vision, but otherwise not a muscle stirred into action. We did consider the idea of some kind of treadmill to make her work for her food, but in the end her charm and her feline physiology had us beat and we reluctantly agreed that she was better fat and happy than thin and miserable.

She has caused some amusing misunderstandings in her time. On one occasion a young representative from a drug company called at the surgery, as they do from time to time. As we walked through from the waiting room to the office, Pudding ambled across our path.

'Oh! Don't mind her,' I told the rep, as he hesitated to let her pass. 'She is only the practice cat!' His face dropped and he adopted an expression of concern.

'What's the problem?' I was forced to ask, unaware of the reason for his upset.

'Oh,' he said, somewhat sheepishly, 'It's just that I didn't know that you practised on cats!'

In his relative inexperience he must have thought that when vets were faced with tricky operations on perhaps an influential client's pet cat, they would first try out their intended surgical technique on their own 'practise' moggy!

Pudding had become not only a fixture at the practice, but something of a celebrity on the telly. Now, she sat on the consulting-room table, comfortable in the knowledge that food was not far away, as I rewound the measuring tape and wrapped up my spiel on the folly of any animal becoming too overweight. Bernie smiled her approval. I sighed with relief at the director's thumbs-up sign and Pudding just thudded off the table and headed for her food bowl.

Holding consultations under the critical eye of the camera is quite a bit different from a normal clinic, but it is nothing like as difficult as conducting a surgical operation in the same circumstances.

Most surgeons are a bit uptight anyway at the prospect of operating, so the added strain of having one's every move recorded on film only serves to increase an already tense situation.

The theatre itself has to be reorganized so that the camera will be able to pick up all the necessary action, without showing too much of the gruesome details, which might make the more squeamish in

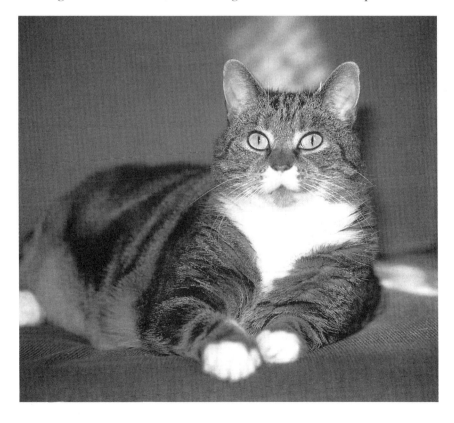

Fat Cat, or Pudding lives permanently at my veterinary surgery and must be the most televised cat in the country.

the audience switch off. Of course, there is no way one can avoid upsetting some viewers. I remember one occasion when I was doing a piece on poop scoopers, I used a plastic replica of a dog's 'jobby' to demonstrate different methods of removing them hygienically and keeping the streets faeces-free! Although my motives were of the highest and in the interests of responsible pet ownership, one viewer did write in to complain. Apparently, he had been having his tea when I launched into my performance.

'I will,' he said, 'never be able to look a sausage in the face again!'

When filming operations, we can never be sure what small detail might be offputting to one viewer or another. Things which may be routine surgery to me could well be distasteful to someone who has a dread of seeing even one drop of blood. For this reason, I take care to select operations which will not be too 'unbearable'.

Lumps and bumps are quite common occurrences in both veterinary and human medical practice, so I thought it might be suitable to feature the many different causes of these in one of my programmes. As with most operations I film, I also have to take whatever patient problem happens to arise around the time we are filming. One of the basic rules of my participation in television is that I will never do or re-do anything just for the sake of the camera. All the work we do on film is still, first and foremost, for the benefit of the patient.

So it was, that I came to operate on Kim Robinson, a black Labrador who was far from being an ideal subject to feature on television. At five years old, he should have weighed around sixty-five or seventy pounds. Kim tipped the scales at a little over one hundred and twenty!

His owner, a lovely old lady, was herself a bit overweight, and when I told her that her dog could do with losing a few pounds, she expressed some concern and vowed that he only had one meal a day! Controlling the desire to inquire as to the size of the pail the meal was served in, I looked at Bernie, and together we raised our eyebrows in disbelief. We had both heard so many owners of obese pets profess the same thing that we could only assume they were motivated by personal guilt. Kim's past history, however, contained details which lent testimony to his desire to eat everything in sight and I considered this more reliable than Mrs Robinson's measure of his diet.

Some weeks previously, the dog had been put out in the grounds of the family home for a bit of exercise and, to make it easier to catch him again, Mr Robinson had left the lead attached to Kim's collar. When the time came to bring the dog in, Kim was sitting contentedly

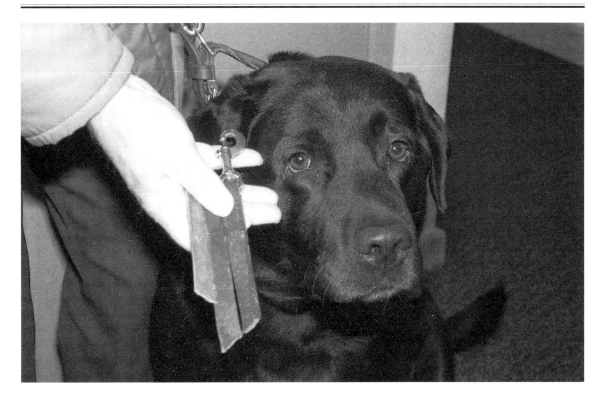

at the door, but all that was left of his lead was the six inches of it attached to the collar itself. It transpired that, after careering round the garden, Kim had felt a bit peckish and, no food being to hand, had decided to eat his own leather lead. All except, that is, the bit he couldn't quite reach!

Luckily, that operation was not one to be recorded in any filming session. Although it was totally successful and five pieces of lead were recovered from Kim's stomach, my struggle against massive abdominal fat deposits was not exactly peak-viewing material.

Now, but a few weeks later, he was back, because he had developed a large lump at the base of his neck. From my experience, I reckoned it was a tumour, so we set up the camera and the lights and got Kim prepared for the operation.

Lying on the table, his excess bulk was even more apparent, and I felt as if my opening words to the camera were being delivered over the brow of a hill rather than from my position behind a patient on the operating table.

With my hands just masking the area, I made an incision through the skin over the lump. Despite the fat lying underneath, I was able to remove the tumour without too much offputting bleeding and only then did I realize what kind of lump it was. As befitted a dog

Kim, a somewhat overweight labrador, has now completely recovered from a stomach complaint, after having an operation to retrieve the parts of his own lead which he had swallowed!

of Kim's stature, the lump turned out to be a lipoma which is the polite medical term for a fat tumour! With the job safely done, I still had to perform the hardest task of all. I had to get the patient off the operating table without giving myself a hernia!

Being overweight is, of course, no laughing matter as it contributes to many medical conditions and, as I have suggested, can greatly increase the risk involved in surgical operations.

One little Dachshund I had to treat some years ago was so fat that the term 'German sausage dog' seemed more than normally appropriate. It was in serious trouble, however, when I diagnosed that it had a foreign body blocking its small intestine. Despite the dog's obese condition the operation had to proceed or it would surely die.

In due course I was able to get the Dachsie anaesthetized and opened up its abdomen. Immediately, great white masses of fat billowed out of the incision and made the location of the obstacle extremely difficult. After much searching I found the site of the obstruction and gingerly opened the bowel with my scalpel. There, to my amazement, was a label looking up at me, with the words clearly printed 'Made in Britain'! Later I was able to ascertain that the label was attached to a tube of glue which the dog had swallowed!

I found it quite funny that a label saying 'Made in Britain' should be found in a fat dog so obviously designed in Germany! Just my luck, of course, that the cameras were not there to capture the moment. Isn't that always the way of things?

Chapter 5

Exceptional Patients

'So how long have you had him, Mr Clark?' Mr Clark lifted his pale bespectacled face from our mutual study of his pet.

'Two years,' he replied, in a rather timid voice.

'And what's his name?' I asked, eager to put Mr Clark at his ease, so that I might better glean some information to aid my diagnosis.

'I call him LG,' he said, now more relaxed in the knowledge that it was his pet and not he, who was under scrutiny. 'I decided on LG because he was light green in colour,' he volunteered without prompting. 'I used to have his brother DG,' he continued, 'but he died.'

'He was dark green then,' I interjected, hoping to impress him with my understanding of his naming system.

'That's right,' he replied, now feeling much more confident that he had picked the right vet for his pet.

I looked down at the beautiful little lacertid lizard that stood, much less nervously than its owner, on my consulting-room table. It was about six inches long, from its nose to the tip of its tail, and its metallic green scales fairly glistened under my examination light. As I checked it over, it cocked its head this way and that, but its sparkling eyes stayed fixed on mine.

'And how long has LG had these warty-like growths on his legs?' I asked.

Mr Clark lifted his dark glasses for a moment and peered at his lizard's legs. 'About six months,' he replied. 'But a couple of other vets I took him to didn't seem interested.'

This rang true. Not many vets were prepared to even look at lizards and other reptiles, far less treat them. I myself had been fortunate to meet a man called Roger Meek, who was not only a fellow Scot but also a herpetologist with an expert knowledge of such creatures. Over the years, Roger the reptile man, as he was known in television circles, not only became a friend, but also taught me all I now know about such species. In return, I would apply what basic medical knowledge I could to any of Roger's own creepy-crawly pets, and together we formed a very worthwhile working relationship. Roger was to become not only my source of reference, but also a valued colleague, when it came to dealing with exotic species on television.

I had long ago decided that it would be folly to try to compete with naturalists like David Attenborough on television. With his access to superb wildlife photography, he could show the viewing public almost unbeatable pictures of the most exotic animals in their natural state. I saw my role as introducing the general public to animals, exotic or otherwise, with problems which could be treated by vets like myself.

When Roger and I were struggling with a four-foot-long Monitor lizard at the opening of one programme, it crossed my mind that David Attenborough had already shown this magnificent animal in the wild. Our lizard, however, had a reason for being on 'It's a Vet's

Roger the reptile man, complete with monitor lizard, explains some of the finer points of herpetology to me and my co-presenter, Marylyn Webb in the studio surgery at Yorkshire Television.

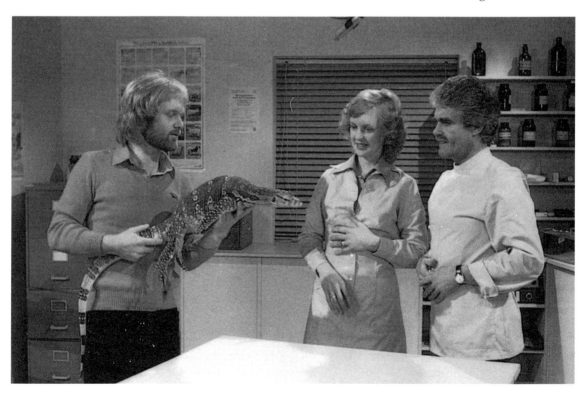

Life' and it showed on the screen. The lizard's large head, with rows of dangerous teeth, was very impressive, but it was the little white bandage round a damaged toe which really caught the audience's imagination.

Over many series, Roger would come on screen and share his wisdom with the viewers and myself, but probably the most nerve-racking time for both of us came when I decided to operate on a Garter snake with a lump on its side.

Roger knew everything there was to know about Garter snakes. He could tell me how they lived, where they lived, what they ate and even what might eat them! What he didn't know was what the lump was and what we could do about it. As a vet, I was well used to removing lumps like this, and often much bigger ones, from cats and dogs. But this snake was not only a completely different type of animal, it was also the first snake I had ever operated on.

'So what are you going to use as an anaesthetic, John?' Roger asked a bit anxiously. It was the first time I had ever seen him uncertain about anything to do with snakes.

'Well, Roger,' I replied, 'the book says Ketamine, so Ketamine it is. You hold the patient and I'll get on with it!'

Roger held the snake, a bit less surely than he normally did, as I slipped the slender hypodermic needle under one of its scales and delivered the calculated dose of drug into the muscle that lay alongside its spine. A few minutes later, the patient lay stretched out almost motionless. I say almost, because Roger, not only an enthusiast but a teacher who revelled in knowledge was at pains to point out that snakes have only got one fully functional lung, and the other is merely a remnant so that any breathing movement is hardly visible.

'If you look closely, John, you can just see the rib cage rising and falling ever so gently,' he said in hushed tones.

'Aye well, you keep your eyes on that breathing, Roger,' I said a bit more abruptly as the tension mounted, 'and I'll get on with removing this lump.'

Roger nodded with the seriousness that such an operation demanded and leaned closer to peer intently at the chest of the sleeping snake.

As I made the elliptical incision around the lump, it felt strange to be cutting through reptilian scales, rather than mammalian skin, but my thoughts on this were superseded by my dismay at seeing such watery-looking blood seeping from the incision.

'My goodness Roger, this snake has got to be pretty anaemic. Take a look at the watery blood.'

Roger unglued his eyes from the snake's chest and in a matter-of-fact voice passed on another piece of his vast knowledge. 'No John, I suspect that will be quite normal for snakes. You see,' he added, focusing once more on the chest and resuming his primary task, 'they have far fewer red cells in their blood than mammalian species do.'

'Thanks Roger,' I said, 'that makes me feel a whole lot better about this patient's chances of survival.' I resumed my work on the lump.

'That's got it,' I announced proudly, as the lump came away. 'Now we can get it off to pathology, and see what it is.' The expected complimentary remarks from Roger on a successful operation never materialized. His thoughts were elsewhere, and the atmosphere in the operating theatre became tinged with anxiety rather than relief.

'It has stopped breathing,' exclaimed Roger, with both urgency and panic in his voice.

'When?' I demanded shortly. At such times words can waste valuable seconds.

'Just this minute,' said Roger, his face a bit ashen with the possibility that he might somehow be blamed.

'All right Roger,' I consoled him, 'don't let's panic yet. Pass me that syringe.'

Almost like an automaton, he did as I indicated.

'Hang on John,' said Roger, 'you know snakes can stop breathing for quite a long time.'

I picked up the limp body of the snake as Roger continued to pour out any fragments of his knowledge which might prove useful.

'And,' he said, 'they sometimes play dead, if they get too stressed.'

'Well, this little blighter has got exactly thirty seconds to stop playing dead or he's getting this,' I said, holding up the micro-syringe which contained a respiratory stimulant. This drug would make the snake breathe if it had a spark of life left in its body.

Roger and I were now both in that unknown territory that lay between the boundaries of our individual fields of knowledge. He looked at my face as if to find the answer there. I reciprocated, but the thirty seconds were up and if there's one thing a surgeon must be, it's decisive. I jabbed in the needle and as the chemical coursed to the snake's nervous system and triggered the muscles of respiration, Roger once more fixed his eyes on its chest.

'There it goes, John,' he announced triumphantly. 'Well done.'

I didn't say anything. I just blessed my good fortune and got on with stitching up the snake's wound. Roger and I learned a lot that day and despite the slight deviation which the wound made to its pattern of stripes, the snake survived.

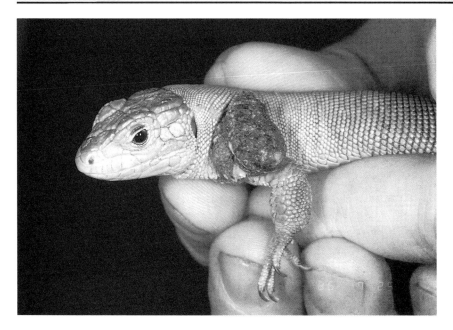

This beautiful green lacertid lizard, called LG, developed a large warty growth on his shoulder.

I picked up little LG in my hand to examine more closely the warty outgrowths which covered almost all of his upper forearm and extended onto his chest wall.

'I'm afraid that it will mean several operations, Mr Clark, and if you don't mind, I would like to discuss your pet's problem on television.' At the very mention of the telly, Mr Clark went a shade paler and stepped back.

'I wouldn't have to be on, would I?' he asked, as if 'on' meant being next for the gallows.

'No, no,' I assured him. 'I would just need to borrow LG and show his warty condition in the morning and do the op in the afternoon.' Mr Clark was only too happy to leave LG and the details of the required surgery entirely to me.

Little LG had several factors in his favour when it came to making the grade for a television appearance. He was an exotic animal and handsome with it. Rarity combined with beauty certainly made him spectacular. Besides that, for appearing on 'It's a Vet's Life', he had that other essential ingredient, a problem I might be able to help with.

It was obvious to me that sharp surgery with a scalpel was out of the question in this case. Even if LG could have withstood the surgical shock, I feared that the unavoidable blood loss would have finished him. Transfusions for green lizards are not yet available! There was, however, a technique called cryosurgery, which uses no cutting at all. This procedure depends on the destructive power of ultra-low freezing temperatures to kill off unwanted growths. It is a bit like controlled frostbite and to produce it, I use liquid nitrogen at minus one hundred and ninety-six degrees centigrade. That's pretty darned cold!

With Charlie and the crew focused in on little LG, I talked about the lizard's problem and the need for surgery. Then, passing LG to Bernie, I went on to demonstrate the basis of cryosurgery for the viewer's better understanding. Arranged in front of me on the table I had a white flask labelled in red with the words 'Liquid Nitrogen'. Beside it, in a wide-mouthed thermos flask, there was some more of this colourless clear liquid. Next to that, a champagne glass with water and a bunch of flowers in a vase. It looked more like a set for science fiction than a surgery consulting room, but after all, this was television and the more spectacular the visual effects were, the better. Cryosurgery is a wonderful technique for both animals and humans alike, and as yet it is not widely enough employed in medicine. Here was my chance to publicize it further.

'In this flask,' I said to the camera, 'is liquid nitrogen at minus one hundred and ninety-six degrees Centigrade. This table,' I nodded towards the one from which I had just lifted the flask, 'is at room temperature, around plus twenty degrees Centigrade.' I hesitated a moment as I undid the stopper from the flask to allow the audience to appreciate better that this meant a temperature difference of two hundred and sixteen degrees! 'Imagine,' I said, 'the effect of pouring cold water into a white hot furnace, that, in reverse, is what will happen when I pour this extremely cold liquid on to this relatively hot table.' So saying, I poured a little of the liquid nitrogen onto the tabletop, where it immediately volatilized into clouds of nitrogen vapour. Charlie had already pulled back to a wide shot as the full splendour of the billowing white clouds enveloped the table, myself and some of the crew.

As the cloud cleared, I picked up the champagne glass half filled with water. 'This,' I told the viewers, 'is unfortunately not champagne, but tap water, again at room temperature.' I poured a little liquid nitrogen into the glass and again the temperature difference caused small waves of white vapour to roll over the rim of the glass in true horror-movie style. 'Magic,' I said, lifting the glass close to my face in the knowledge that it would make a nice close-up for Charlie.

'But seriously folks,' I continued, 'this freezing capability of liquid nitrogen can be put to a very valuable medical use. Watch,' I invited the viewers, as I picked a flower from the vase. 'This is living tissue. It is soft and flexible,' I added, bending the petals and the stem to make my point. 'Now watch closely what happens when I immerse it in liquid nitrogen.' As I spoke, I gently introduced the flower head into the flask. Immediately the liquid nitrogen in the flask boiled into life and the now expected white waves of nitrogen vapour cascaded over its rim across the table and onto the floor. Within seconds, the rushing noise ceased and the vapour subsided. 'Now look at this,' I said, picking the flower out of the flask. 'Because of the extreme cold, it has been completely killed off. It is now brittle and porcelain-like.' To demonstrate, I snapped off a petal from the frosted flower which still gave off a wisp of vapour.

'If this flower head were a growth, ' I looked intently into the camera lens to stress the point, 'it would be completely destroyed.' As I spoke, I slowly and deliberately grasped the frozen flower head in my hand and crushed it. 'Gone for good,' I said, as I slowly sprinkled the glass-like fragments of the crushed flower head onto the table and held up the stem.

Later that afternoon, the cameras recorded a different and more serious theatrical scene, as I used some sophisticated equipment to deliver the liquid nitrogen to the affected areas and freeze off little LG's warty growths. In the editing suite at Yorkshire Television, the whole thing would be put together to form not only an entertaining piece of television but one which might also introduce the audience to a new and sophisticated surgical technique.

LG lived to tell the tale and even appeared on future programmes to sport his wart-free exterior before the cameras.

The smaller a patient is, the greater the risk often is. Nevertheless, vets must be prepared to operate on all sizes of animals if it is in the patient's best interests.

Long before television came into my life, I had fashioned the principles by which I would work within my chosen profession. The most important of these was my determination never to do anything with an animal unless it was truly in that animal's interest. In order to adhere to this, I always ask myself 'What would I want if I were in that animal's place?'

One day, across my consulting-room table, I was faced by a well-dressed lady holding the hand of her seven-year-old daughter. She had just placed a small cardboard box on the table.

'This is Nicola,' she said, glancing down at her daughter, who gave a little smile in response, 'and this,' she said, tapping the cardboard box, 'is Dixie her pet mouse.' Nicola's smile blossomed at the mention of her pet's name. 'Tell the nice gentleman about Dixie's little problem,' urged Nicola's mother.

Love for an animal has got little to do with size: when a young girl's pet mouse developed a breast tumour it was a very serious matter.

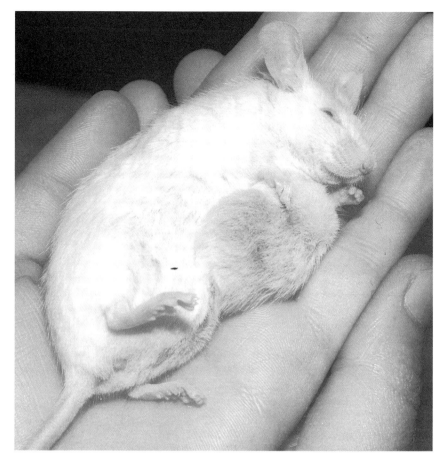

'I want you to make Dixie better,' said the little girl, looking directly into my eyes.

As I picked up the box to open it, her mother surreptitiously caught my eye, and with a knowing look, shook her head silently from side to side. 'Play along!' her expression told me, 'but there is really nothing that you can do.'

'Well let's see,' I said, opening the box and leaning down towards Nicola. 'Is Dixie a nice wee mouse?' I asked, as Nicola's eyes opened wide and her smile said everything about her love for her pet.

'Oh yes!' she said in soft sincerity, 'Dixie is the best mouse in the world.'

As I lifted the little white mouse from the box and gently turned it over, I could see that it had a large growth on one of its breasts. 'Have you seen this?' I asked, turning the mouse's underside towards mother and child. Mother looked a little sadly at her daughter, and then back at me. Again and out of view of Nicola, she shook her head at the hopelessness of it all.

Little Nicola looked up at me with her big brown eyes. 'I know,' she said, acknowledging the lump, and then in the innocence of her childhood, added, 'She'll need a hoperation won't she?'

'I looked across at her mother who shook her head even more meaningfully. If I had stressed the risks and the slim chances of survival, or even suggested a replacement mouse, I know of no person who would have held it against me. But then, there were those two brown eyes and Nicola's childlike belief that I could make her Dixie better.

'Tell you what, Nicola,' I said, 'you leave your little mouse with me and I'll see what I can do.' Nicola smiled warmly up at me. She had faith that little Dixie was in good hands.

'I'll do my best,' I told the mother quietly as they were leaving, 'but I can't make any promises.'

'I know, I know,' she whispered back, shaking her head again. 'It looks hopeless.'

'Give me a ring about lunchtime tomorrow,' I said, showing her out, 'and I'll let you know what happened.'

Nicola left full of hope. Her mother left convinced she would never see Dixie again. To be honest, the odds in my medical mind favoured the mother's position.

With that little white mouse anaesthetized and laid out on the operating table, the lump if anything, looked larger. With its tiny

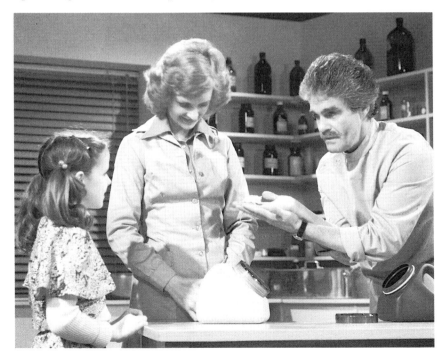

Nicola tells the story of Dixie's successful operation, in the studio.

legs taped out with sticky tape to hold it on its back, I started the operation. On a larger animal like a dog or a cat, the operation can be tricky. In one as small as a mouse it might well be impossible. Despite the difficulties, I did get the lump off with the minimum of blood loss and stitched up the wound with suture material generally used for delicate eye operations.

'Okay Bernie,' I said, 'all we can do now is hope that the surgical shock isn't too much for it.'

Bernie took the wee mouse and, returning it to its cardboard box, she cocooned it in a warm covering of cotton wool. She then placed the box in the surgery incubator.

'Just come and see this,' said Bernie, poking her head round the stairs as soon as I had finished my batch of afternoon consultations. I followed her up to the recovery room and was amazed to see a totally awake Dixie, not only out of her box, but clambering all over, checking out her new incubator home.

'Better keep her in there all night, Bernie,' I said, overjoyed at Dixie's recovery. 'If we control the temperature for the next twelve hours, who knows?' I crossed my fingers and Bernie smiled back at me sympathetically.

Needless to say, Dixie not only survived the op but went home the next day to a delighted Nicola, who knew all along that everything would be okay. Mother was not only amazed, but declared the whole affair a miracle.

The real miracle, of course, had more to do with a young girl's faith that something could be done, a faith that had made an ordinary vet and his nurse try to do it.

A week later, I received from seven-year-old Nicola the best letter of my life. From the style and the writing used, I could tell that her mother had had no hand in it, but to this day, I still have that letter and use it from time to time to remind me that miracles are possible.

'It must be lovely,' wrote Nicola, 'to be able to hoperate on animals as small as a mouse and have them come through. Dixie can't talk so I'm writing for her. Thank you a million times. Love, Nicola.'

All that happened many years ago, and I suppose that Nicola will now have more interest in men than in mice, but I often wonder if she realized how important she and little Dixie were, to the future path taken by this practising vet.

Chapter 6

On Location

I sometimes have a tendency, both as a vet and a television presenter, to bite off slightly more than I know I can chew.

'So, have we got everything we need, Bernie?' Bernie my veterinary nurse and right-hand man in all things medical, nodded.

'The only thing I'm not a hundred per cent sure of,' she added ruefully, 'is the safety of that container of liquid nitrogen.'

I had wedged the cryostat containing about twenty-five litres of liquid nitrogen on the back seat of the car, and made it doubly safe by putting a seatbelt around it.

'Don't worry, Bernie. It is quite secure.' I reassured her, as I double checked its stability. The last thing we wanted, as we headed into the Yorkshire countryside was the car awash with liquid nitrogen at minus one hundred and ninety six degrees centigrade.

That morning we had arranged to meet the film crew and a lady vet called Carol Paterson, at the farm of one of her clients. In our never ending search for a variety of venues and animals for 'It's a Vet's Life' this was to be one of our 'down on the farm' locations. The journey, through the country roads of Yorkshire, was a pleasant change from my usual city surroundings, and we arrived at the farm to find the crew already busy, checking out the situation and deciding how best to shoot the piece for maximum impact.

The main subject of the filming was to be a magnificent grey horse who had unfortunately developed multiple growths on a very delicate part of his body. I had volunteered to remove them by cryosurgery, but first we had to get the horse under an anaesthetic and that was most definitely a job for Carol. She may have been a lady vet of slender proportions, but when it came to handling animals, she was a real toughie. With her broad Scots accent and a

A piece about a special jacket that prevents hypothermia in lambs was a nice introduction to the work of farm vet Carol Paterson.

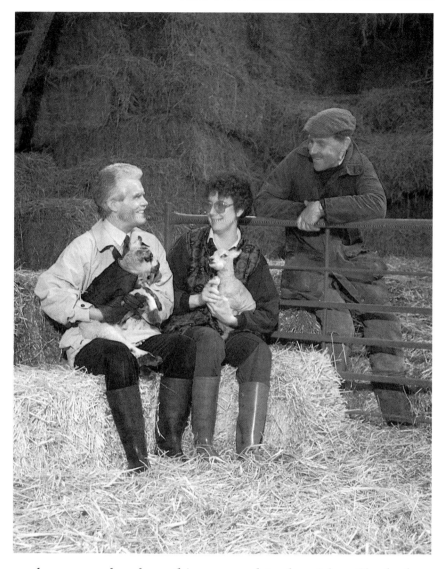

ready raucous laugh, nothing seemed to daunt her. She had an outgoing, ready for anything personality that is made for television and together we not only produced some good material, but had a whale of a time doing it.

I had worked with Carol a couple of times before on other programmes in the series and on one of these occasions, she took on the mammoth task of putting a new ring in a Hereford bull's nose. One look at the huge beast in its stall was enough to make me thankful that I was a pet vet, but for the diminutive Carol, it was all in a day's work.

'Just you stand back, John,' she advised me. 'Until the stockman and I get him into the crush.' I didn't need a second telling as she and her helper prodded and cajoled the great bull into the metal-framed crush, and secured his head by locking a hinged bar against the side of his neck.

'Okay John,' she laughed, 'you can come back now.'

Standing next to the massive head of that magnificent beast, I could really appreciate the enormity of its size and its awesome power.

In my student days, I remember seeing a country vet, and well remember his advice.

'Never get anywhere near a bull,' he told me sternly 'unless he has been properly restrained.'

He should have known, because he had learned the hard way when a bull had accidentally crushed him against the wall of a cattle shed and ruptured the muscles of his abdomen. He had six months in hospital to contemplate his folly and was in no hurry to have it happen to anyone else.

Carol's bull was well restrained and from my close viewpoint, I could now see the excessive wear on the ring it had in its nose. If the pull on this tender part of his anatomy was to continue to be effective in leading him, then a new ring would have to be fitted, and that was a job for Carol.

'Try and steady his head for me, John,' she instructed with professional authority in her voice, 'while I saw aff this auld ring.' I noted that Carol had slipped into the Scottish dialect with her 'aff this auld ring,' and appreciated that I did just the same in my moments of tension.

I grasped the bull's head as best I could, as it snorted its hot breath down gigantic nostrils, at the indignity of the whole affair. Strong as any bull he might be, but the skill and ingenuity of a slender lady vet had him by the nose. Carol's breathing accelerated as she sawed away at the old ring, and being a gentleman and a vet, I felt I should offer to lend a hand.

'Och aye, help yourself,' agreed Carol cheerfully, and added 'You know, sometimes we can undo the wee screw that holds the ring together, but this one's got a bit corroded.' I hadn't even seen the screw, far less decided it was corroded. I thought that they all had to be sawn off. A couple of minutes later and the job was done. The 'auld' ring was out and Carol, quick as a flash, produced a brand new shiny one. This, she hinged open and fed through the existing hole in the bull's nose and then clicked it shut.

'This is the screw,' she said, as if she'd known all along, that I hadn't noticed the corroded one, and she deftly located it and screwed it home. 'There you go son,' she said, patting the bull on his broad curly forehead and releasing the retaining arm of the crush. 'I hope that didn't damage your male pride too much!'

By the look in the animal's eye and his defiant snort as he backed out of the cage, I doubted if anything could dent his masculinity!

On another occasion I had seen how farm vets, ladies or not, have to have a fair degree of physical strength if they are to carry out some aspects of their job.

The director had suggested that dehorning a cow might make an unusual item, especially with a lady vet doing the job. Naturally, Carol was favourite, and this time it was a cow and not a great bull that stood before us with its head secured in the crush cage. Dehorning dairy cattle is quite a common procedure and is done so that they don't damage one another in the intensive bustling environment of a modern dairy farm.

'If you just hold her head round, John, I'll slip a wee injection of local anaesthetic in at the base of the horn.' This time my task was a little more feasible than with the Hereford bull. I grabbed the cow's nose with the fingers of one hand, and the horn with the other and twisted its neck round with all my strength.

'That's fine John,' Carol complimented me. 'Now just change sides and I'll inject the other horn.'

Once the anaesthetic had taken effect, Carol produced a very large bone saw and set to with gusto. I could see the effort she was putting in and made a professional decision not to interfere. She was, I excused myself, used to this kind of work, and after all I was a pet vet, who was certainly not used it. The first horn came off with hardly a drop of blood and, confidently changing sides, I spurred Carol on to finish the job on the remaining horn. This time, just as the saw had nearly severed the second horn at its base, the farm hand who held the halter to keep the cow's head round, let it slip.

One moment, I was an interested observer watching the work of a lady farm vet and interpreting it for the viewing public, as any self-respecting TV presenter should. The next, I was leaping back in a frantic panic as two jets of arterial blood from the base of the severed horn hit me full on my immaculate pale blue anorak, and sprayed me from head to foot.

'Och, you'll be all right, John,' said Carol, as she casually clamped the bleeding vessels and twisted them off with artery forceps. 'The farmer's wife will soon have you spick and span again for the telly!'

True to her word, Carol whisked me into the spacious farm kitchen where a rosy-cheeked farmer's wife in a floral apron apologized for the trouble that her husband's cow had caused a 'star' like me. Then, she proceeded to peel me out of the blood-soaked anorak and, rinsing it through under the cold water tap, popped it into the oldest electric washing machine I have ever seen. As Carol and I tucked into cake in the kitchen, the machine vibrated violently as it beat the bloodstains from my coat. Dried and pressed like new in twenty minutes, I was ready for my next immaculate piece to camera and the viewing public would never know what had gone on 'behind' the scenes'.

Today's job was one with two major differences. The first was that Carol wasn't going to do the job this time; I was. And, the other was that I hadn't yet seen the growth which the horse had on its private parts.

One of the problems with farm animals and wild animals alike, is that it is sometimes difficult even to get a look at the source of their trouble. Perhaps that's the reason I became a pet vet! In such cases, restraint becomes a top priority, and with this horse it was going to take anaesthesia.

'So how are you going to knock him out?' I asked Carol, hoping that she would have a ready answer.

'Well John,' she replied, 'that all depends on how long your op is going to take.' Carol was a shrewd lady and knew the wisdom of answering one question with another.

'That depends on how big the growth is, Carol,' I replied. 'But I reckon that it will take about half an hour.'

'Right then,' she said, in her customary matter-of-fact manner. 'I'll give him a shot of sedative to quieten him and then knock him down with thiopentone.'

Carol busied herself with syringes and bottles, and by the time Bernie and I had garbed ourselves up in our green surgical gowns and lugged the container of liquid nitrogen from the car, the horse was lying on its side and sleeping peacefully. With ropes on the horse's hind feet, the horse owner and her friends were co-opted to position the legs so that I could get a look at the problem, and what a problem it proved to be!

Inside the horse's prepuce and extending onto the surface of its penis, there were multiple black growths, each about the size of a walnut. Even Carol was a bit dismayed.

'Are you going to be able to do anything for it, John?' she asked with real concern in her voice.

'We can only try, Carol,' I replied, and coupled the long flexible pipe to the liquid nitrogen flask and fitted on a spray nozzle.

Faced as I was with such a surgically difficult task, all thoughts of how it would look on television became secondary. In this situation, I am a veterinary surgeon first and a television presenter a very poor second. Fortunately, the small crew who have worked with me for years are just as professional as I am, so as Bernie and I struggled to destroy the tumour, they moved tactfully around the 'scene' to record the sound and pictures that would make an impressive item for the programme.

As the jet of liquid nitrogen was played over the tumour masses, large clouds of white nitrogen vapour formed around the operating area to give the whole scene a surrealistic appearance.

My estimate of half an hour was well out. By the time I had frozen all the tumours, the anaesthetic and my surgical stamina were well-nigh exhausted.

'Did you get any of that?' I asked Charlie. He nodded with the reverence that operations often instil. Of course he had, I thought. I may have performed the operation but he and the rest of the crew would shape the story and make it work on the television screen.

Two days later, Carol was on the phone in a panic. 'John, I know that you said it would swell a bit, but you should see it. It's gigantic!'

I could tell by the urgency in her voice that the swelling must have been spectacular. Carol was one calm lady. I had never heard such alarm in her voice.

'Okay Carol,' I tried to sound as reassuring as I could. 'You always get some swelling after cryosurgery. It's just an effect of the extreme cold. It will go down, trust me.'

'I hope you're right, John,' she answered, now sounding slightly less apprehensive, 'because it's some swelling. How long do you think it will take?'

'How is the horse itself?' I parried, hoping to glean more information.

'Och, he's fine. He's eating well and everything, but John,' she couldn't help herself saying it, 'you should see the size of his "willie".'

'Look Carol,' I said eager to help 'give the horse a shot of steroid and let me know how he is tomorrow.'

As Carol rang off, I could imagine the scene at the farm as the young owner and her family and friends questioned the wisdom of letting a pet vet loose with his new fangled cryosurgery on their beloved horse. I could see them gathering round the patient, pointing at his massively enlarged private parts and expecting the worst. Luckily, I knew that although there might be some swelling, the horse would have no pain or bleeding and all I had to do was to retain my stature as the 'expert' and keep my cool.

The next day, Carol rang to report that the swelling was still large but going down. At the end of that week everything was back to normal size and the owner and the family had regained a little of their faith in the veterinary profession. Four weeks after the operation, Carol reported that all the tumours were now gone and that the horse was in fine fettle and best of all, she asked if I could send some autographed photographs for the owner and her family.

Ah well, if you want to portray the real aspects of a vet's life, you have to let the cameras in on ops like that. My only regret is that I didn't get Charlie back to film the post-operative swelling. It would have made a spectacular piece of television but I doubt very much if many of the viewers could have stomached it on the screen!

Chapter 7

Sensitive Problems

As must be clear by now, holding a surgery for the sake of the television cameras is a completely different affair from my everyday consultations as a practising vet.

'Don't look at the camera at all,' I advised Mrs Walsh, as she fidgeted with the string of expensive pearls around her neck. 'Try to imagine that you and I are just talking together about Toby's problem, and that the crew and the camera don't exist.'

Mrs Walsh nodded nervously and over-patted her spaniel who sat unconcerned on the table in front of us. He couldn't care less that he and his problem were about to be discussed and recorded on film for all to see. To give the impression of a normal consultation, and the future audience a feeling that they are getting a privileged view of something which is usually very private, I started the item by examining Toby's eyes, ears and mouth. This gave Charlie, the cameraman, a chance to start with a close-up of the dog's head and then pull back to reveal the wider shot of me talking to Mrs Walsh with Toby on the table.

'So how long have you been having this rather personal problem with Toby?' I looked directly into Mrs Walsh's eyes and launched this section of the programme which was intended to deal with pets' sexual problems.

'Oh, it must be about two or three years now,' answered Mrs Walsh with a niceness tinged with naïveté.

I had been a little concerned that this might not be an appropriate subject for the series. However, if anyone could talk about the matter in a genuine and sincere way it was nice Mrs Walsh.

'So what did he get up to first?' I coaxed her into her story, as

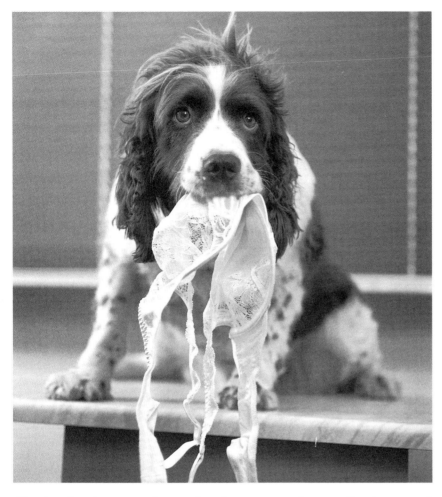

When Toby the spaniel got a trifle over amorous it became a little embarrassing for all concerned.

Charlie slowly zoomed in on her face to record every fleeting mood and expression.

'Well you know, at first he would only grab my leg like young dogs do, and sometimes have a go with a cushion,' she blushed almost imperceptibly, and continued, 'and then he started to follow me all over the place.'

'Understandable,' I reassured her. 'Toby was your dog. You loved him and he loved you.' Mrs Walsh nodded enthusiastically. 'But,' I encouraged her, 'he just took things a bit far, didn't he?'

Mrs Walsh warmed to her tale and, giving Toby a little hug, carried on. 'Yes he did, Mr Baxter. He started following me into the bathroom when I was taking a bath and then he would make off with bits of my underwear.' I had visions of Toby grabbing a pair of Mrs Walsh's pants or perhaps her bra and making off up the garden to bury his trophy like a favourite bone.

'He never chewed them up or anything,' she went on, 'he seemed to just want to sniff at them.'

As a vet, I could see the reason for Toby's behaviour all too clearly. People have pets to share love and loyalty, one with the other, but the combination of Mrs Walsh's loving nature and Toby's canine machismo had brought things to a point where embarrassment and inconvenience had introduced a little disharmony into their relationship. There is nothing wrong with signs of sexual attraction, but they have to be at the right time, in the right place and with the right 'person'. Toby was only showing a very natural need for sexual expression but it didn't fit in with the social niceties of being a domestic pet.

'Does Toby's behaviour upset you a lot?' I asked.

'No,' came the almost immediate reply, 'but my husband and my friends get a bit bothered by it.'

'Ah well, no need to worry,' I said, 'because there is a drug which I can inject into Toby and perhaps reduce his male hormone response and so cool his ardour. If that works, we can make the effects permanent by castrating him if you wish.'

Mrs Walsh looked slightly taken aback by the severity of the solution and even when I explained that the operation would only remove his sexual drive and not alter him in other ways, I somehow felt that she was not entirely convinced.

'Cut,' said Charlie, not to reinforce my suggestion but to terminate the interview. Toby looked a little uncertain and leaped from the table.

One of the valuable features of a medical programme like 'It's a Vet's Life' is the opportunity it affords the viewers to witness a confidential situation 'through the keyhole' as it were. Since many of the problems are associated with the alteration of private bodily functions, this makes the privilege all the more interesting.

The lady who came in next had what she considered to be an urgent problem with her pet hamster. After my usual advice about ignoring the camera, I realized that no amount of calming chat was going to settle this lady down. Camera or not, she wanted an answer to her pet's medical problem.

'It's my hamster Harry,' she said, hoisting the fat wee furry creature, still half asleep, from the midst of his cotton wool comfort.

'What's the problem?' I interjected, keeping my fingers well away until I had established that Harry was both fully awake and reasonably good-tempered. Hamsters are not averse to sinking their very sharp teeth into any prodding finger, friendly or otherwise and there is a well-told story in veterinary circles about a vet and a hamster. With the best will in the world, this vet picked up his hamster patient and poked at it with a diagnostic finger in an attempt to find out what ailed it. With the speed of a striking cobra, the previously comatose hamster returned to life and sank its teeth into the vet's index finger. Despite the spurt of bright red blood, the hamster continued to hang on to the finger for dear life. The vet, not surprisingly, reacted to the sudden pain and almost by reflex shook his hand vigorously to dislodge his clinging attacker. This may not have been a trained professional action, but it did have the desired effect, even if the end result was disastrous.

The offensive hamster was not only shaken free, but hit the hard floor of the consulting room with such force that the patient's original problem lost all significance. Despite recovering his cool and being abject in his apologies, the vet not only lost a substantial amount of blood but also most of his professional reputation. The distraught owner left with her dead hamster and later reported the vet for disciplinary action to the Royal College of Veterinary Surgeons.

Whilst on this subject of dead hamsters, may I digress for a minute to caution anyone who is ill-advised enough to buy one as a pet. Do take special care if one day it appears to be inexplicably deceased. Hamsters, you see, have another capability which they switch on when their body temperature reaches a critical low. At such times, they go into a soporific state, where their little bodies go stiff and immobile and, to all intents and purposes, they appear dead.

Not all that long ago, I had a letter from a lady in Ireland who had heard me mention this 'sleeper' condition in hamsters, when I was a guest on 'This Morning' for Granada Television. Apparently, little Steven, her grandson, had found Henry his hamster lying dead one morning and was very broken up at the loss of his pet. His father not only sympathized with his son, but promised to buy him a new hamster that very day. Dad then did the expected thing and buried the hamster with due reverence in a selected spot in the garden.

On the way down town to the pet shop, father and son stopped off at grandma's and naturally told the old lady about the sad death of Steven's hamster.

'Are you sure he was really dead?' asked grandma.

'Don't be daft, of course he was dead,' said dad, a bit disgruntled.

'Well,' said the old lady, undaunted by her son's admonishment, 'I just saw a vet called John Baxter on "This Morning" with the Madeleys and he said that all dead hamsters should be...'

Her son cut her short with an even sterner rebuke. 'Look, Mum,' he said, 'you don't think I'd be stupid enough to bury a hamster that wasn't dead! I think you'd do better to stick to your knitting!'

The old lady shook her head, confident that what she had heard on the telly had to be the gospel truth. Dad, in mild indignation, left with his son to buy the new hamster.

Picking the pet replacement was no trouble at all, but Steven and his dad arrived home to find Steven's older brother standing on the doorstep. He was in an excited state to say the least.

'You know Henry your hamster,' he cried out to Steven, as they came up the path. 'Well,' he stammered, 'he has come back to life.'

Dad, with grandma's words still ringing in his ears, stared in disbelief, but then there was no denying what his eyes could see. There, clutched in his older lad's hands was indeed little Henry, looking none the worse for having survived not only death, but burial that very morning! Apparently, the next-door neighbour had spotted Henry emerging from the freshly dug soil of his grave, where he had eaten his way out of his cardboard coffin and tunnelled to the surface. None the worse for his interment, Henry seemed much less perturbed by his return from the dead than Steven's father was!

'The lesson to be learned,' I explained to the viewing audience, when not only myself but Steven and his miraculous hamster appeared on 'This Morning' a couple of weeks later, 'is to make sure you warm up any apparently dead hamster on a hot water bottle before deciding to bury it!'

The hamster which the anxious Mrs Hudson now held in her hands was very much alive and as she upended it to make her concern even more evident, she said pointedly, 'You see, Doctor, the poor wee thing has got cancer.' She looked straight at me, biting her lip with worry. Forgetting my concern over the flashing front teeth, I took the hamster from her overly tight grasp.

'Whereabouts?' I asked, failing to see any obvious signs of such a serious condition.

'Just there,' said Mrs Hudson, scarcely able to conceal her irritation that a qualified vet could not see the problem. She pointed a red-lacquered nail towards the hamster's nether regions. There, sure enough, were two large swellings. 'These two growths,' she said, jabbing again with her finger. 'It's cancer isn't it? Is it going to kill him?' she asked with real concern.

'I doubt it very much, madam,' I replied with as little sarcasm as I could. 'You see, these two lumps are his testicles!'

As the light of realization dawned on her, the embarrassment somehow made her resent my superior knowledge, and she hurried

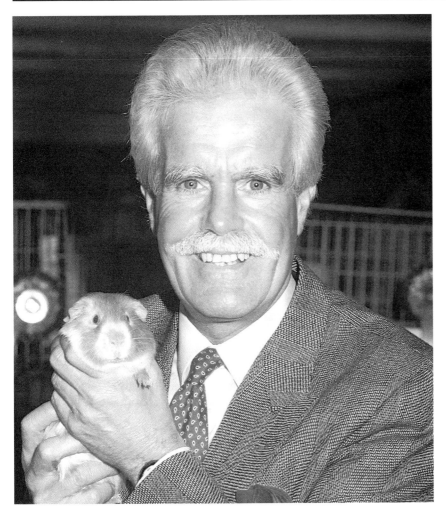

A guinea pig patient, whose supposedly sensitive problem was diagnosed as being perfectly normal.

blushing from my surgery. If only she had known that, a few days previously, I too had shown just such an ignorance of normal anatomy with another of my clients.

This particular lady, in an attempt to distance herself from the delicate subject of sex, but unable to contain her curiosity, had contacted me by phone.

'My guinea pig,' she announced with the confidence of obscurity, 'has got a growth on the end of its private parts.'

I hesitated, as one does when confronted by a gap in one's own knowledge or experience.

'Is that right?' I asked inanely. 'And what does it look like?'

'Well,' she replied warming to the intimate nature of the problem, 'it's got two kind of horn things...and they wave about. Do you think it has a growth?'

'To be truthful,' I replied 'I can't say I've ever been confronted by such a problem before. Bring the guinea pig to the surgery and let me have a look.'

Not many minutes later, the lady, with a suitably serious expression, arrived at the surgery and solemnly produced the guinea pig from a cardboard box. As she held it up by the shoulders, I gently probed between its back legs and, at length, managed to extrude its little pointed penis. To my surprise and the owner's obvious delight, there confronting me, was the strangest structure I had ever seen. Two little horns, for all the world like a miniature version of the bull horns that adorn the cars of Texas cattlemen, waved their presence towards my unbelieving eyes.

'Well,' I told the lady, 'I haven't a clue what they are, but by the look of them, I would say they are part of the guinea pig's natural equipment, rather than growths.' So saying, I sent the lady off, half satisfied, with a promise that I would find out more.

That afternoon, I contacted a lady who devotes almost all of her waking hours to the welfare of guinea pigs and must surely be one of the world's foremost authorities on these animals.

'Ah yes,' she replied, when I cagily presented her with the problem. 'These are perfectly normal in the male guinea pig, and they are called "keratinaceous styles". A pretty name for them, don't you think?' she remarked.

'I think that you had better spell that for me,' I said, and having written it down, thanked her for the information and rang off.

'Have you got that now?' I asked my guinea-pig client, having imparted my new-found knowledge to her, and then added, 'and don't forget to tell all your friends about them at your next coffee morning!'

Mind you, if she does discuss it with her friends, she might be called upon to explain how she came to be looking at her guinea pig's willie in the first place!

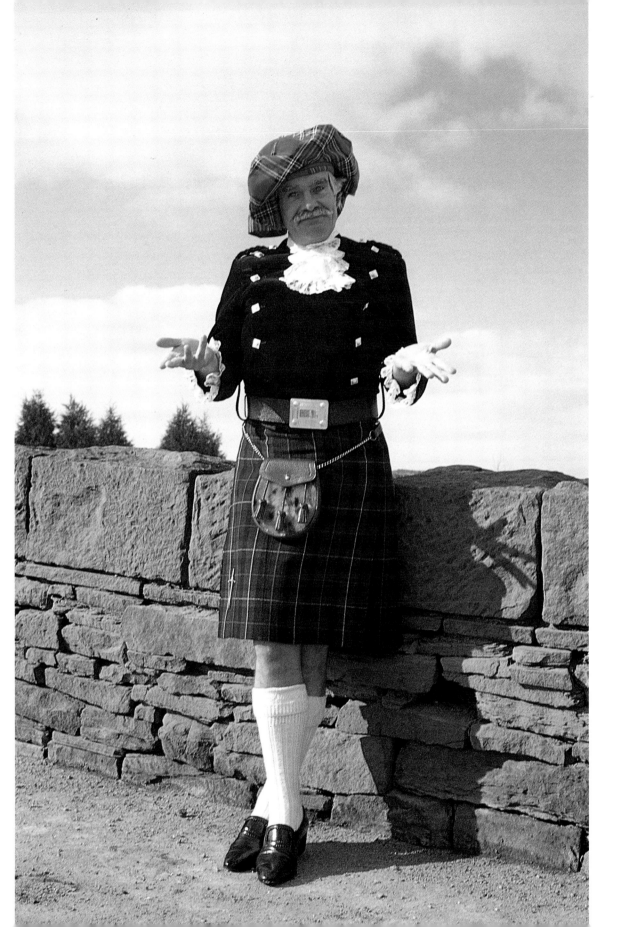

PREVIOUS PAGE: Highland attire may be a real eye-catcher but it can get a bit draughty during a Scottish winter.

RIGHT: 'Fat Cat's' reason for appearing on screen is not to achieve fame and fortune, it is for that extra bit of food in her dish – after the filming!

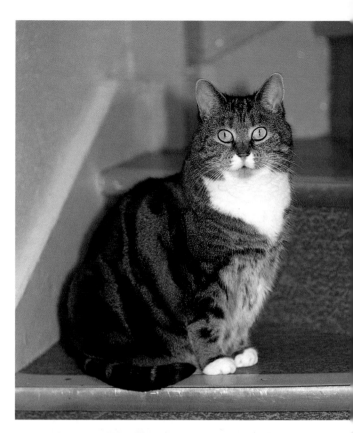

BELOW: Geoff Hughes showed a softer and more caring side of his character, and displayed his love for country life, when he brought one of his pet lambs on to the set of 'It's a Vet's Life'.

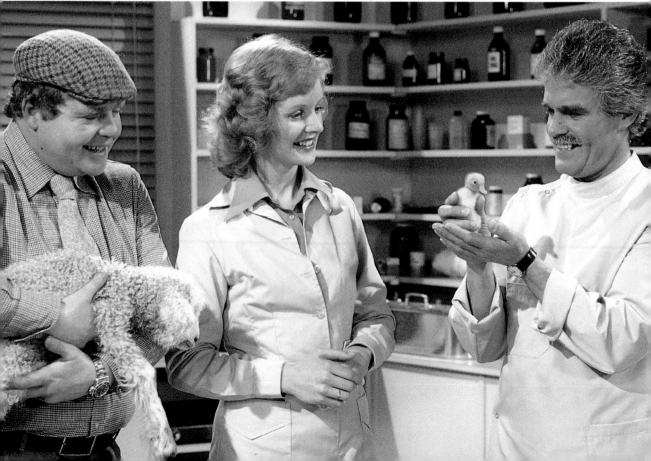

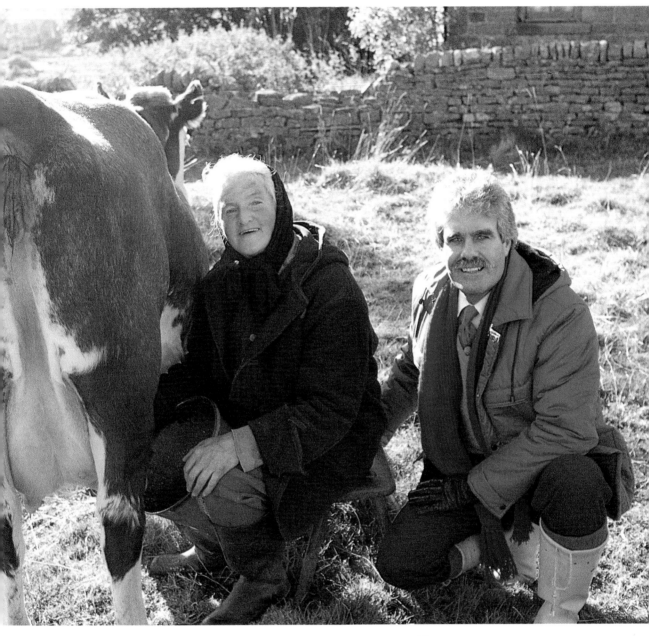

On location at the isolated hill farm owned by Hannah Hawkswell. We were able to film a little of the challenging lifestyle of this unique and remarkable lady.

Peaches the kitten was born without a proper bottom and was close to death when he was brought to my surgery.

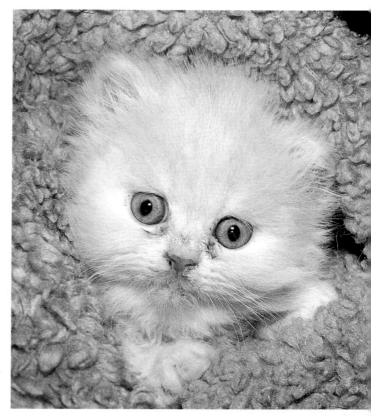

It would take more than a urinating tortoise to dampen the enthusiasm of Judy and Richard, the two polished presenters of Granada Television's 'This Morning'.

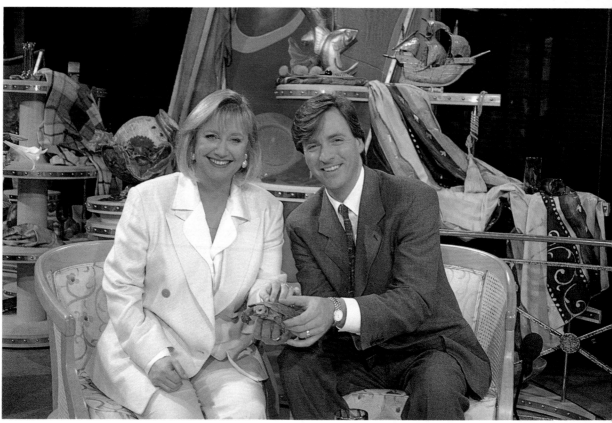

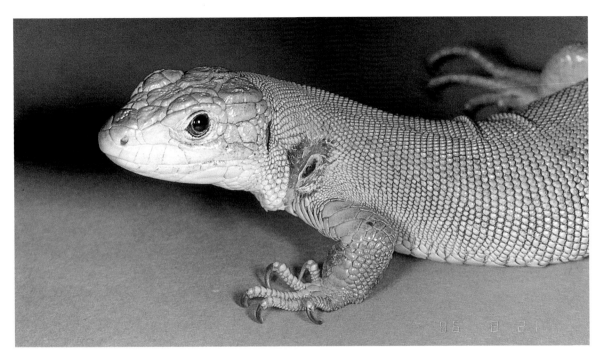

ABOVE: LG, a beautiful green lacertid lizard had a large growth removed thanks to the technique, cryosurgery. He was left with only a very small scar to show where it had been.

BELOW: Seals, with their large and attractive eyes are appealing at any time, but in the caring atmosphere of the crèche in Pieterburn, Holland, they seem even more so.

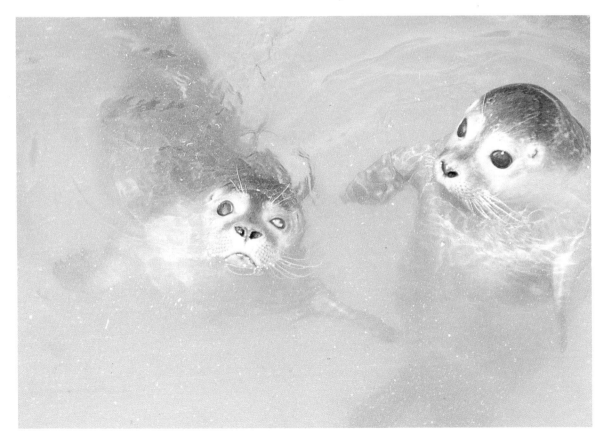

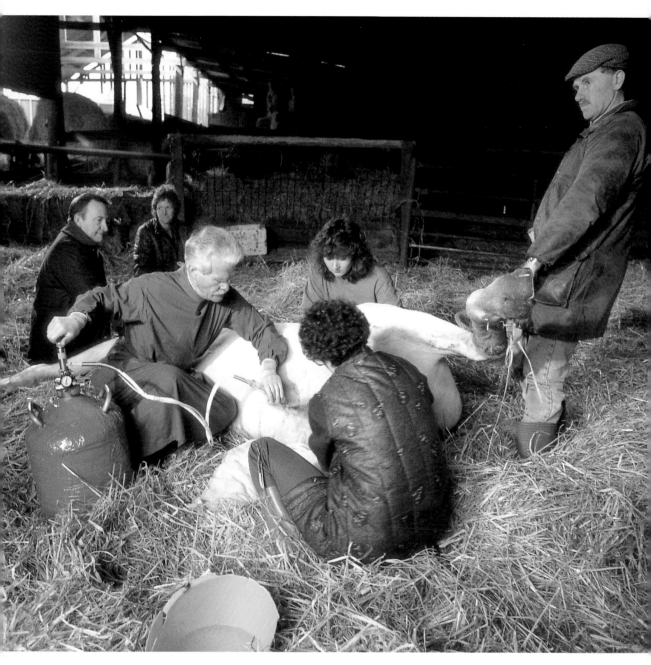

Operating on a horse 'down on the farm' proved to be a bigger job than I expected.

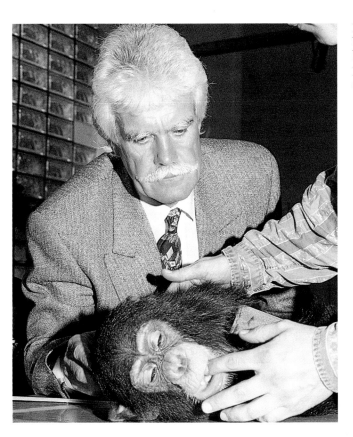

Fast asleep under a general anaesthetic, a baby chimp is about to undergo a whole battery of medical tests. Later during post-operative filming, he managed to get his own back!

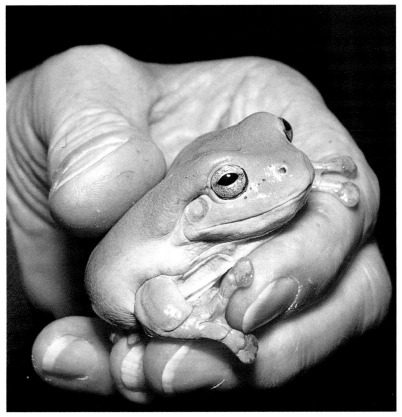

This spectacular green frog was not only attractive, but also quite a long jumper, as a certain young BBC presenter found out when it landed in his lap.

Roles get a bit reversed when my co-presenter, Gaynor Barnes takes me for a Singapore spin in a pedal powered rickshaw.

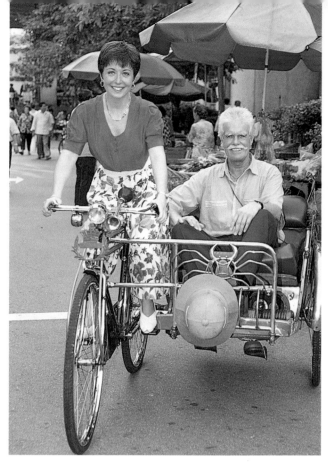

John meets up with an amiable Orang-utan at Singapore Zoo, when filming the 1994 series of 'It's a Vet's Life'.

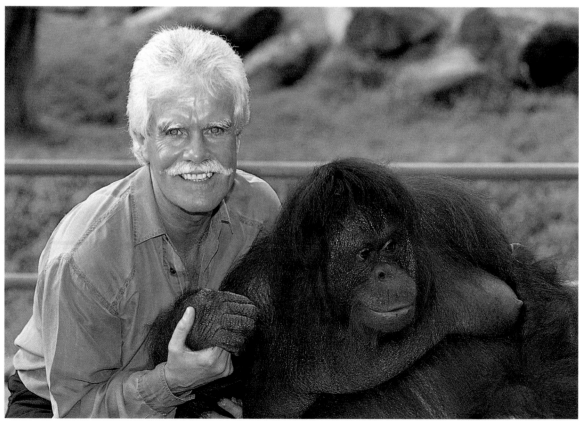

Chapter 8

Going to the Zoo

The great tiger spat and snarled his discontent, as the two keepers prodded him along the caged walk towards us.

The zoo vet and myself stood back as the big cat was half-forced, half-enticed into the small purpose-built cage in front of us. A metal door clanged shut behind the tiger and despite his power, the ingenuity of man now had him confined in this narrow space.

'Okay,' said Nigel, one of the London Zoo vets. 'Just let me get him crushed against our side of the cage, and you will be able to give him that injection.'

As if he understood our intention, the tiger turned his massive head towards me, curling back his lips and flattening his ears to his head. Then he let out a roar that had my hair standing on end and every fibre in my body screaming at me to flee.

'Some teeth, eh?' said the smiling zoo vet spotting my look of panic. 'It's certainly just as well we've got these steel bars between him and us.'

I swallowed hard and smiled back, having already taken in every detail of the tiger's massive fangs. The zoo vet then pulled a long lever and a metal partition on the far side of the tiger's cage moved towards us. The tiger instantly sensed the meaning of this action and roaring his defiance, fairly shook the whole contraption in his futile efforts to escape.

'I hope the lad who designed this cage used strong enough steel,' I joked with Nigel, who was busy drawing up the sedative solution into a hypodermic syringe.

'High-grade, John,' he replied. 'These bars could hold back an elephant.' I welcomed his confidence, but knew that I would feel even better when this great cat was sound asleep.

Apparently the tiger had been seen by one of the keepers to be limping badly on its right foreleg. The zoo vet had been called in to find the reason. A frequent problem in dealing with any sick or injured animal is getting its permission to examine it. In my surgery with dogs and cats for patients, I am generally very fortunate. They are all domesticated pets and will allow me to conduct a thorough examination and even take blood samples whilst they stand patiently on my consulting-room table. As a rule, wild animals won't allow a vet anywhere near them, far less permit a stethoscope on their chest or a thermometer up their bottom. Any examination that has to be done either has to be conducted visually from a distance or when the animal is under restraint. This may simply mean a trusted keeper being able to physically hold an animal in his arms, or much more commonly, as with this non-cooperative tiger, the administration of a sedative injection to put it to sleep temporarily. This is not always as straightforward as it might seem!

My old friend, Tom Begg, who studied with me at Glasgow University, did become a zoo vet when he qualified, and I had occasion to visit him when he was professionally associated with a private zoo in the south of England. He told me about a problem he had just experienced when he had to give a young chimpanzee some medicine.

'I knew,' Tom told me, 'that there was little point in trying to give the young chimp his medicine off a spoon as you would a human child. Chimps are not only very clever, they are also very suspicious. 'Sometimes,' he explained, knowing how little knowledge I had of working with zoo animals, 'we have to try and disguise the medicine in something else. Ribena is often a good cover-up for baby chimps but this latest lad I had to treat was too wily for that. I decided that I had to be a bit more cunning and a bit more scientific than any chimp.

'What I did was to get a banana and inject the medicine inside it using a syringe and a very fine needle. Of course, I did this well out of sight of my chimp patient. These chimps, you see, are so clever that if you open the banana without them seeing you do it, they won't touch it. So,' Tom continued, 'I got the young chimp and after a few minutes of cuddling and playing around to give him confidence, I produced the doctored banana and offered it to him. He took it eagerly, but just sat in the safety of my arms and did nothing with it. "Go on then, eat it up," I coaxed, using my free hand to mime the peeling of the banana.'

Tom could hardly believe his luck when the little chimp followed his bidding and deftly peeled back the skin from the top half of the banana. Then, once again, he just sat there with the half-peeled fruit in his hand and looked at Tom as if waiting for further instructions. Tom's keen scientific eyes had already scanned the surface of the peeled banana for any tell-tale signs of his previous interference. It looked perfectly normal, not even a needle mark.

'Go on then,' said Tom, intimating the next phase of his plan, by opening his own mouth and pointing an index finger into it repeatedly.

It was of course Tom's intention that the chimp should now eat the banana, but whether by smell or some other sense, the young animal realized that all was not well and instead, he followed Tom's directions to the letter, and rammed the banana into Tom's already open mouth! It was fortunate that the medicine was only a simple antibiotic and not a strong sedative like we were about to give to this ferocious tiger.

The zoo vet passed me the syringe. 'I thought that you might like to give it the jab, John,' he said with a smile. 'After all, you'll be quite used to injecting cats in your own surgery!' True enough I had injected pet moggies every day of my practising life, but they were made more tolerant by domesticity than this raging beast in the cage before me.

'Great,' I said, taking the syringe, 'I would love to have a go. Shall I put it into the muscle of his back leg?'

'Yes, John. The back leg will be fine and it will keep you as far away as possible from those teeth!'

I glanced at the head end where the tiger showed his displeasure at the whole affair by fixing me with ferocious eyes and spitting his defiance. Even crushed against the cage side, the tiger did his level best to avoid being injected and it took me a couple of attempts before I got the needle soundly home. All we had to do now was to wait patiently for the drug to have its effect.

In the noise and excitement I had forgotten all about the fact that we were filming the whole thing, but a casual nod from the director told me that he already had all he wanted.

'If you grab the front of the stretcher, John, I'll take this end,' said Nigel, 'and we'll get him to the operating theatre.' Gone were the snarls and spitting, all that remained was the soft snoring of a tiger at rest.

On the examination table, the vet quickly diagnosed that the tiger's lameness was due to a wrist injury and, after x-raying the joint, he left me in charge as he went to the next room to process the x-ray plate.

Lying sedated on the table, the tiger still looked magnificent, and I decided that this was too good a television opportunity to miss. The way to do it, I decided, was to compare this tiger with an ordinary domestic cat. I picked up one of the tiger's massive paws and after explaining its wrist problem, I unsheathed one of its razor-sharp claws and explained that it not only had killing weapons on all four feet, but also in its mouth. To illustrate this last point I lifted the tiger's great sleeping head and tilted it towards the camera. As I did so, I must admit to wondering if it would stay fully asleep, particularly since the zoo vet who knew about such things was still nextdoor! Undaunted, I opened its great jaws and pointed out its long dagger-like fangs. That was the cue for the whole crew to take off, out of the op theatre and down the corridor.

Taking chances for television was all part of their stock in trade, but confronting male tigers who might just wake up at any minute, was pushing their professionalism a bit too far. Thankfully, the brave cameraman stuck to his post and we were able to record one of the most memorable moments I have ever experienced at any zoo.

Perhaps the only one that comes close, was when we were filming recently at Amsterdam Zoo. In the course of taking some general views in order to set the scene, Charlie decided to shoot some footage of the gorillas. These wonderful primates had private quarters opening out into a communal play area which had hillocks and tree stumps to give such intelligent animals an interesting environment. This whole outside area was surrounded by a strong circular plate-glass screen, which gave the public ideal viewing conditions.

During his filming of these animals, Charlie asked the sound man to put the end of his mike, which was on an extending pole, over the top of the glass barrier to collect some realistic and natural sound. This is what the professionals call 'nat sof', an abbreviation for 'natural sound on film'.

Ian duly extended his pole until the grey windproof mike could just reach across the top of the glass and poke into the compound. He was not to know that in the animal kingdom, that was an uninvited intrusion and totally out of order. The public's place was outside the glass barrier and inside was strictly gorilla territory.

Most of the group of gorillas, both young and old, looked at Ian as if he was the worst person on earth, but one middle-aged male decided that more definitive action was called for. Both Charlie and myself had spotted him before this episode and from his permanently disgruntled expression and bellicose attitude, it was clear that he had a massive chip on his shoulder even before Ian decided to violate his personal space.

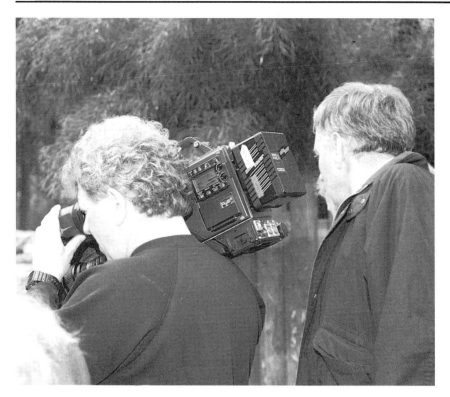

Cameraman, Charlie, and sound engineer, Ian, intent on capturing all the action in the gorilla enclosure at Amsterdam Zoo.

As Ian, under the threatening gaze of the group, edged his mike back to his own side of the glass, the bad-tempered male took off from the summit of a hillock and threw himself bodily at the glass. The smack of the resulting impact and the roar of his protest sent all of the crew and most of the public spectators scampering backwards for their dear lives. The angry gorilla headed back to his hillock with a 'that will show you' swagger and adopted his usual grumpy expression. During the course of the next few minutes, it became clear to Charlie that Ian was the primary cause of this crotchety gorilla's current displeasure. Re-positioning the sound recordist close to the glass, Charlie asked my co-presenter and myself to sit on the small wall that formed the base for the glass barrier.

'Get ready to go when I tell you,' he said.

With our backs to the glass we could see nothing of what was going on behind us, but Charlie obviously could. As Ian moved closer to the glass, Charlie had one eye on the camera eyepiece and the other on the grumpy gorilla. At the moment he decided appropriate from the primate's expression, Charlie signalled us with a whispered, 'Action,' and I sallied forth into my introduction.

'Today, in "It's a Vet's Life" we have come,' I said, 'to Amsterdam Zoo in Holland.' My co-presenter was then supposed to come in

Taking off as an angry gorilla smashes into the glass screen behind me. This was a great example of reflex action and was most definitely not in the script!

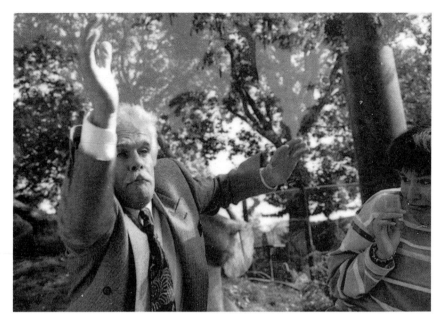

with her bit, but just as she was about to start, the gorilla scurried across and once more launched himself at the glass!

The rest was down to adrenaline and reflex action as two previously cool and professional TV presenters took off like a couple of rockets. Never in my life have I had such a fright or moved with such speed, but the resulting film footage made it all worthwhile. If Charlie had told me what he was planning, I would have given very good odds against his ever getting it on film. However, thanks to a bad-tempered gorilla and an imaginative director with a high degree of skill, we managed to record a memorable bit of television. To this day, Ian the sound man is not so sure it was all such a good idea!

These unexpected bits of 'luck' always help lift any section of location filming and we were doubly 'lucky' at Amsterdam Zoo when I had to do a piece to camera with a baby chimpanzee who was about to have an operation. Crouched down in a public viewing area, surrounded by a multitude of Dutch parents and their children, I held the cuddliest of baby chimps in my arms and it was very easy to think of the words I wanted to say to the camera.

'Well,' I said, 'I've seen and held some wonderful animals on "It's a Vet's Life" but surely none could be more charming or attractive than this baby chimp.' As I said this with the conviction of true feeling, I felt the flow of warm liquid hitting my right thigh and running down my leg. Realizing that the little chimp had just relieved itself, I added, 'which has just peed on me!'

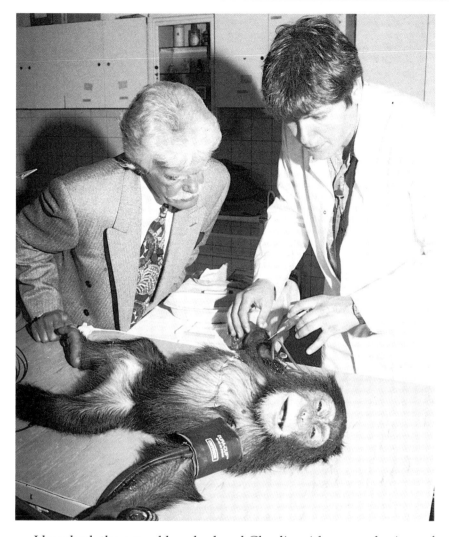

Operations such as this make fascinating viewing, particularly when the patient is as adorable as this baby chimp.

I laughed, the crowd laughed and Charlie with a superb piece of intuitive camera work tilted the lens down to record the urine dripping onto the concrete floor and then he swung the camera back on to me giving the wee chimp a cuddle of forgiveness.

Despite these 'magic moments', which, incidentally, made their way on to 'It'll be Alright on the Night', my attitude to zoos has always been a bit ambivalent. On the one hand they do a lot of useful work, not least on behalf of endangered species, but I have always felt that behind all this, there is a profit-making motive which is built on selling the spectacle of unusual animals to the public. Perhaps showing people wild animals on film whilst they are still actually in their natural wild environment would be a much better idea than containing them in the unnatural setting of zoological gardens.

On a recent visit to Singapore where we were filming for 'It's a Vet's Life' one of our locations was Singapore Zoo. Here, apart from presiding over an efficient and well-run establishment, the zoo director had come up with a novel and exciting concept. His idea, in my estimation, makes a welcome compromise between the inherent restriction of zoos and the freedom and dangers of the wild. What they are now offering at Singapore Zoo is a totally new attraction called 'Night Safari'.

'The majority of wild animals,' Bernard, the zoo director, told me, 'are nocturnal, and when we look at them during the day they may be sluggish or sometimes even asleep. So,' he continued, 'we have been building for several years now a whole new "jungle" area, which will allow the public to see wild animals in a much more realistic and natural state than in any other zoo.'

What they have done is to encompass an area of natural jungle and to divide it up for different groups of animals. Each section has been replanted where necessary to match the differing requirements of each species and, where segregation is essential, it has been done using concealed moats and barriers rather than fences. Experts in all the many fields needed for such a venture have come from all over the world, and not least of these has been the British specialist who designed the lighting. Strategically placed in the trees, concealed lighting filters down to give a most realistic appearance of a moonlit night.

When the project is wholly completed, people visiting the zoo will be able to go on specific walks through the park at night or take a more leisurely trip through this jungle setting on an electric buggy.

When Gaynor, my co-presenter, and I were given a sneak preview, I really wasn't prepared for the impact that the scene would have upon me. As we and a group of VIPs cruised silently in convoy through the jungle we 'came upon' groups of animals behaving much more naturally than I had ever seen them do before. It was as if we were the visitors in their rightful territory rather than the more common situation where they are contained in ours.

Long-legged giraffes browsed gracefully over the trees and mountain sheep skipped nimbly from one rockface to another. It was, however, the antics of three young tigers which made the most lasting impression on me. Only twenty feet from our buggy, they played a cat and mouse game with each other in the jungle forest as I am sure they would have done, learning how to kill, in the wild.

This was indeed a far cry from the caged cats I had seen in my youth at far-off Edinburgh Zoo, and if it makes a happier life for zoo animals, then I am all for it.

Chapter 9

Back-end Bother

'What do you think, Mr Baxter?' asked Mrs Cowlishaw, with concern in her voice. She held out a tiny underweight white Persian kitten towards me. 'Can we do something for her?'

I looked down at the scraggy little thing and knew instinctively that it had already been lucky to survive this long. 'How old is it?' I asked, as the kitten opened its mouth and meowed pitifully.

'She's only four weeks old,' she said, knowing as well as I did that the kitten was so small it might have been only four days old.

Mrs Cowlishaw and her two daughters were dyed in the wool animal lovers and their devotion to their dogs and cats was carried to such an extent that some might have considered them eccentric, if not downright foolish. Not that anyone else's opinion would have

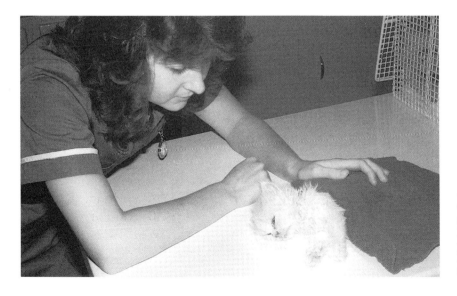

After a long and tricky operation to reconstruct a new exit for his bowel, Peaches sleeps peacefully under the loving care of Bernie, the nurse.

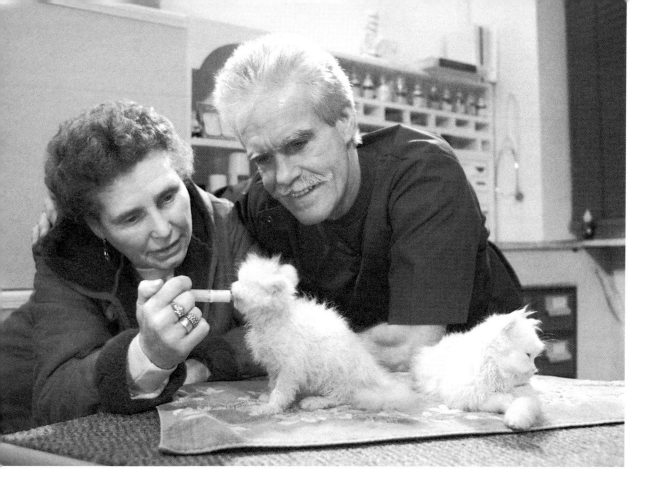

The love, devotion and not least the hard work of Snowball's owner, were key factors in saving the life of this tiny kitten.

made the slightest difference to the Cowlishaws. They loved their pets and that was all there was to it!

'I can't make any promises, Mrs Cowlishaw,' I said cautiously, knowing that the odds were stacked against the kitten's survival, 'but if you are willing to take over the nursing and bottle feeding I shall be happy to do what little I can.'

One of Mrs Cowlishaw's daughters, warmed by the slightest prospect of the kitten's recovery, emerged smiling from behind her mother. 'We don't mind staying up all night for a month if it means saving little Snowball, do we mum?' Mum nodded, but she and I knew the prospects were not good.

It was going to take a miracle and not only were miracles hard to come by but Mrs Cowlishaw had already had one the previous year. Two miracles in two years is a bit much for even the most zealous of animal-lovers to hope for.

The last 'miracle' had involved another Persian kitten called Peaches. Peaches was only a few days old when Mrs Cowlishaw had brought him in to see me as a last resort, as two other vets had pronounced it a hopeless case. The kitten's belly was distended and it was obvious that he was in quite a bit of pain. The reason, which

Mrs Cowlishaw in her experience had already guessed, was that Peaches had been born without a proper bottom. He had no exit from which to empty his bowels. That explained not only his discomfort and abdominal distension but prophesied an early death if the fault could not be corrected. The risks of surgery were great in so small a patient, but there was no alternative.

'I trust you, Mr Baxter,' said Mrs Cowlishaw, turning to leave her precious Peaches in my care. 'If anyone can save him, you can.'

With little Peaches anaesthetized and lying asleep on an operating table designed for much larger pets, I wondered if I would be able to live up to Mrs Cowlishaw's confidence in me.

'I've never seen anything like it,' I confided in Bernie, as I stood scrubbed-up and in my green operating gown ready to go.

'Well,' replied Bernie, a master of milking every ounce of skill out of me in difficult situations, 'I know you will do your best.'

'That's for sure,' I replied, and set to with the most miniature instruments in my possession. Using equipment designed for eye surgery, but ideal size for such a mini patient, I eventually managed to correct the defect and re-establish an artificial exit for the bowel. In effect, I had made Peaches a new and functional bottom.

After the two-hour op, as little Peaches lay recovering under a warm blanket in the incubator, I felt somehow confident that he was going to make it.

'Well done, Mr B,' chirped Bernie, with a lightness in her voice which further bolstered my confidence in the eventual outcome.

It transpired that we had to operate another three times in the ensuing months to enlarge the opening as Peaches grew to adulthood. It was, however, a testament to Mrs Cowlishaw's determination, and to her faith in me, that later that year a fully grown and spectacularly beautiful Peaches made his television debut just before little Snowball's sad appearance on the scene.

Now, another little Persian was fighting for her life, but this time I knew, for certain, that her owners would give their all to save her life. This time the struggle may not have involved the delicate surgery that was used in Peaches' treatment, but the little kitten's struggle for survival made compulsive viewing.

With artificial milk administered from a miniature feeding bottle, little Snowball struggled through several weeks of nursing and treatment before learning to eat and drink for herself.

With her progress being recorded each couple of weeks or so, the viewers were kept up to date, and when the cameras finally recorded Snowball's first few unaided laps from a saucer of milk, there wasn't a dry eye in the surgery.

Drama, I have discovered, is not only created by spectacular events but is often embodied in the little things that accompany the everyday struggle for existence. Either our own or that of 'someone' we love.

Mr and Mrs Myers had no children of their own, but had given their love instead to a family of three lovely German Shepherd dogs called Zoe, Cassie and Ballou. Over the years I had treated all of them for a variety of medical and surgical conditions, but now the only one of the 'babies' still alive was the youngest one, Ballou.

When she fell ill, with her most recent complaint, the signs were at first quite subtle.

'She sometimes stumbles, Mr Baxter, and seems to trail her back feet a bit,' replied Mrs Myers, in answer to my request for information. 'I hope I'm not wasting your time,' she said. 'It may be something or nothing.'

'Just let me have a look at it,' I replied, picking up one of Ballou's rear feet and looking at her nails. There, sure enough, were the telltale signs of her trailing her feet. The top of the nails were worn down by being dragged over rough abrasive surfaces.

'Does she have any trouble getting up from a sitting position?' I asked, nudging the dog's hind quarters and watching her overcorrect her balance.

'Yes she does, Mr Baxter, and I've noticed,' she added, 'that she sometimes wobbles a bit on the back end as she walks.'

'Well, I shall have to x-ray her to see how bad or good her hips are,' I advised Mrs Myers, 'but I am already pretty sure that she has a condition called CDRM.'

I went on to explain that CDRM was an abbreviation for quite a mouthful of a medical condition called Chronic Demyelinating Radiculo-Myelopathy. Unfortunately, no one as yet knows the cause of this condition and even worse, there is currently no known treatment.

'What will happen to Ballou?' asked Mrs Myers, concerned for the welfare of the last of her 'babies'. 'Will she be in pain?'

'No,' I replied confidently, 'that at least, I can promise you, but she will get progressively more and more disabled until, eventually, she will become totally paralysed.'

'So I won't have to have her put to sleep?' asked a somewhat relieved Mrs Myers, using an expression for euthanasia often employed in the veterinary world.

'No Mrs Myers, you can keep her as long as you and your husband feel able to support her,' I told her. 'It will be no different from looking after a disabled person, but I must warn you now,' I added, feeling it only fair to do so, 'they often become incontinent and it can mean an awful lot of work.'

'Oh, I don't mind the work,' retorted a remarkably cheerful Mrs Myers, 'and Mr Myers is big and strong and can help me carry her outside whenever she needs to go.'

Ballou did pretty well for almost two years, but eventually her disability advanced so much that her rear legs were practically useless. She could, however, still pull herself around at a remarkable speed with the power of her front end! When she came into the surgery, Paul would grab her rear legs then lift her off the ground and run her in, wheelbarrow-style, for a check-up.

Of course the incontinence, which was now complete, did make an awful lot of work for Mr and Mrs Myers, but they seemed to take it all in their stride. As long as Ballou was not in any pain, they wanted to persevere. I must admit, I would not have blamed them for taking an easier way out, but I was both proud and pleased that they had chosen to struggle on.

When faced with such dilemmas in my professional career, I always ask myself, 'What would I want if it were me?' In Ballou's case, I would want to go on, especially with such loving and willing parents as the Myers were.

Ballou's case was a tragically sad one, but it did prove that a vet's life is not all cures and successes. Like all of medicine it has its fair share of failures and disasters and I talked over the possibility of featuring CDRM in one of the programmes with the producer. Together, we felt that the story, treated the right way, could be a valuable addition, not only for the series, but for veterinary medicine in general.

Charlie, the director, decided on a change of set and positioned Mrs Myers in the waiting room with Ballou lying at her feet. My co-presenter, Gaynor, a lovely girl with a caring and sensitive attitude, started off the interview. I had already explained in a previous piece to camera what CDRM was, and now it was up to Gaynor to fill in the viewing public on what it meant to own a dog with such a crippling condition. In response to Gaynor's questions, Mrs Myers managed to paint a graphic picture of how she coped with a disabled and incontinent dog.

'I use nappies, just like you would for a baby,' she said. 'When we know she needs to go, Paul and I sometimes manage to carry her outside.'

It was, however, when Gaynor sympathetically broached the subject of whether Mr and Mrs Myers had ever considered 'putting Ballou to sleep' that Mrs Myers broke down. Until then, her composure was, if anything, only marked by a little tension and a whole lot of love for her dog. Now her pent-up emotions surfaced in tearful sobs and Mrs Myers broke down completely, apologizing for letting the television crew down.

I looked at the producer, and he nodded for me to move in. I put a reassuring arm round the tearful Mrs Myers and gave her a big hug.

'Come on, now,' I said cheerfully, 'or you are going to have me crying.' That was actually closer to the truth than anyone knew.

Mrs Myers mopped up the tears and laughed with me. After all, we had been through a lot together with her Ballou and this was only for a TV programme!

'Hey,' I said, trying to keep the atmosphere a bit more upbeat, 'have you ever thought of trying one of these?' I then brought up into shot, with my other hand, a miniature version of a contraption which is used for supporting the paralysed rear end of dogs.

'This one,' I said, 'is designed for a much smaller dog than yours, but if you care to give it a go, I have managed to borrow a full-sized German Shepherd version for Ballou to try.'

Of course, I knew Mr and Mrs Myers would be happy to try out anything I might suggest, if they thought it would help their beloved Ballou.

'Right,' I said, to Mrs Myers, nodded agreement, 'I shall get the wheels in motion and get hold of that canine wheelchair for your dog.'

Charlie and Mike were, of course, well aware of the filming possibilities, but what none of us knew was whether Ballou would even tolerate being strapped into this canine cart, far less trundle around happily in it.

So it was arranged to meet the Myers a couple of days later, and together we all trooped off to the local park. I must admit that I was more excited about the prospect of Ballou's performance than about any I had previously made on the screen.

Ballou was in due course lifted from the car by Mr Myers and walked wheelbarrow-style down the grassy incline to the footpath that encircled the park itself. There, on the tarmac surface, he and his wife soon had Ballou's back end suspended over the wheel structure and strapped into place over the cushioned pads. Almost before Charlie could get the camera onto his shoulder, Ballou was off. For the first time in years she felt the freedom to move around, sniff at other dogs' calling cards, and even turn full circle to see what was keeping Mr and Mrs Myers, who were now trying hard to keep up with her!

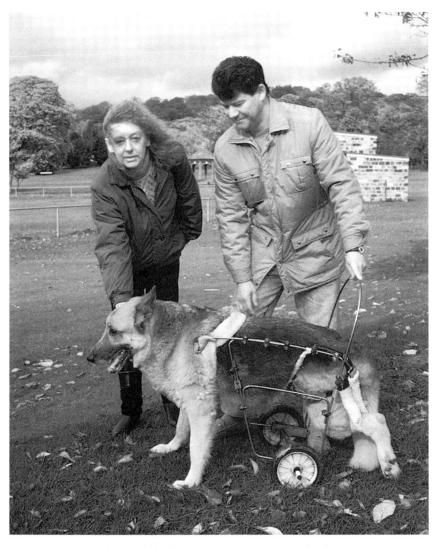

It is not all that common to see a disabled dog in a wheelchair, but as well as helping the dog to lead a more active life, it persuaded a wealthy businessman to fund research into a crippling disease.

As my vet's heart filled with emotion, I watched Mrs Myers give her husband's hand a wee squeeze of proud self-satisfaction to see her 'baby' make such a successful second go of walking under her own power.

I doubt if there will be many such satisfying episodes in anyone's life, and I would certainly hate to have missed that slightly unusual scene of a very caring couple and their disabled dog out for a walk in the park!

If any icing were needed on such a splendid cake, may I finish by recounting a related story which started perhaps halfway through the Ballou saga.

Because of my interest in CDRM and its effects on Ballou and others of my German Shepherd patients, I had tried to do what I could by writing about the condition, as well as airing it on the telly.

Down south in Essex, a wealthy retired businessman noted my interest, and since his own beloved German Shepherd dog, Rebel, had died from the very same condition, he approached me and asked where he might invest a substantial sum of his money to help fight this crippling condition.

'You could do no better,' I told him with confidence, 'than give any grant you might decide, to the Veterinary School at Glasgow University. They have there, the best team of vets in the country.'

I admit that I was a bit biased, being both Scottish and an old boy of the very same Veterinary School. I was impressed by their reputation before I went there. I was impressed while I was studying, and what is most important of all, I have remained impressed throughout my career as a practising vet. With some academics at some university establishments one can easily get the impression that they see themselves in an ivory-towered environment and react accordingly. On more than one occasion, I have had the distinct feeling that I am trying to converse with some hot-house specimen of a specialist, rather than as one vet speaking to another. This has never been so when I have sought advice from any of the Glasgow team. From my first contact with the telephonist right up to the Dean at the top of the academic tree, they are all so very down-to-earth and eminently approachable.

I remember one occasion when, because of my TV exposure, I was invited to the house of some local wealthy business people, who were holding a special do because a friend of theirs was touring the country to publicize her latest book.

Later, it transpired that their friend was the very famous Barbara Taylor Bradford, and it was on her insistence that I was invited in the first place. I was soon to find out why! Barbara, after getting over the run-of-the-mill chitchat that ladies of her fame have to indulge in, quickly collared me, and got down to the real reason for having me there. Apparently, her beloved Bichon Frise dog, which was back in New York, had suffered a severe slipped disc, become partially paralysed and was in great pain.

'John,' she exclaimed, in genuine concern for her dog, 'I know that you're an expert. Can you perhaps explain things to me? I can't make out what these American vets are trying to tell me. Do you think little Gemmy will be alright?'

It was very obvious that at that moment, Barbara's books and perhaps quite a few of her friends, could have gone out of the window, if only little Gemmy could be okay. Like many less famous

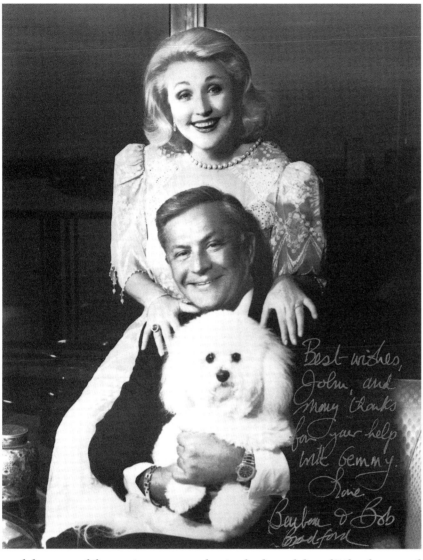

When her dog Gemmy fell ill, bestselling authoress, Barbara Taylor Bradford put her pet before her books and did everything possible to aid Gemmy's recovery.

Best wishes, John, and many thanks for your help with Gemmy. Love. Barbara & Bob Bradford

and less wealthy pet owners, she truly loved her little dog, and wanted to do all she could to help her.

I sat down and with the aid of a pen and paper, I sketched out the simple anatomy of the spine and then set about explaining how a disc can be forced out of place and so put pressure on the nervous cord.

'Depending on the severity of the disc lesion,' I told her, as she listened intently, 'the patient may only feel a transient pain or if it is really bad, he or she could be totally paralysed and incontinent.'

Clearly relieved at being better informed on her dog's general condition, Barbara agreed to phone me each night after she had had her daily contact with the American surgeons at the hospital in New York, where Gemmy was a patient. Barbara's maid supplied the background material whilst Barbara, on my instructions, wrote down everything the American vets reported to her, so that I might translate it into understandable language.

Every night at around ten, my phone would ring, from wherever she was in the country, and Barbara would read off the medical jargon for my interpretation. All went well until some of the technical developments baffled even me and would have only been understood by another neuro-surgeon. That's when I got on to Professor Ian Griffiths at Glasgow Veterinary School.

The upshot was that between us we made Barbara more informed, a lot happier, and what is most important, more able to make informed decisions about what to allow her American vets to do.

In the end, it was well worthwhile, and little Gemmy not only lived but recovered well enough to fairly skip up the steps to Barbara's luxury penthouse flat in New York.

Now a year later, it was the very same Professor Ian Griffiths who would be heading any team investigating the probable cause of CDRM.

Before many months had gone by, I received the good news that a cheque for £100,000 had been donated to the Glasgow Veterinary team and that a four-year study into CDRM was about to be launched.

Wouldn't it be wonderful if the generosity of a businessman, stimulated by something I said on the telly, resulted in a dedicated team of Glasgow vets finding out the cause or even learning to prevent such a dreadfully disabling disease as CDRM?

Now that really would be a worthwhile by-product of any television programme!

Chapter 10

Weird and Wonderful

Television people tend to have seen and done most things, so if you are to stimulate them at all, or even stir their emotions, you have got to come up with something pretty unusual.

As an 'in front of camera' person, I have come to recognize that a true sign of quality in my performance, is when the crew actually gets involved with what I am saying or doing. If I can get them to laugh out loud, I really know I'm on to a winner! After all, the crew is just a very specialized part of my audience, and what works for them will work all the better with the general viewing public.

This became all the more apparent while I was doing one of my many guest appearances on Granada's 'This Morning' programme with Judy Finnigan and Richard Madeley. I was to have a short lead-in chat with these two well-known presenters, introduce a few different animals, and then use this as a 'teaser' for a phone-in later on in the show.

On the large set at the Albert Dock in Liverpool there were not only several pre-set interview areas, but an abundance of technical staff milling about. Compared with my show and its five man crew, 'This Morning' seemed a much busier production.

On one occasion I passed Richard a very unusual type of tortoise, which was one of the rarest species in the world. It had the added distinction of being flat rather than helmet-shaped, and possessed a soft shell rather than a hard one. Possibly because of this last feature, it had also developed the ability to run at high speed! Unlike other species of tortoise, it could take off at a fair rate of knots, find a crevice in the nearest rocky outcrop and then inflate its flattened body so that it became wedged and immovable. This prevented it from being dragged out and eaten by one of the many predators around. As if all of this were not enough to make it television-worthy, this flattened reptile went under the descriptive name of the pancake tortoise!

'Have a feel at its soft shell?' I leaned across and offered Richard the animal. Richard, in true professional style, took it and held it straight in front of him for the cameraman to get its pancake profile in close-up. All of this was great television. An unusual animal, the rarity factor, an unexpected feature in its track record, and also a bit of a funny name. The crew and the Madeleys were obviously intrigued. Then that little bit extra occurred, which brought the house down and made it a memorable piece of television.

'Yes, it's soft,' said Richard, as he held the pancake tortoise up and gently pressed its shell. Just then the animal decided to empty its bladder, and a greater volume of urine than anyone could have believed possible flowed down on to Richard's lap. This may not have endeared the tortoise or myself to Richard, but the crew fell about laughing and I knew the viewers would love it.

Richard returned after the break with trousers duly dried out and we went into the phone-in. Upstairs, a team of tremendous phone-in ladies whose office door is labelled 'The fabulous nobodies' had already taken in excess of two and a half thousand calls on animal problems. These covered all aspects of animal behaviour, from a dog who kept sniffing up ladies' skirts to a cat who insisted on doing her toilet in the houseplant pots. There was even a lady who had a pot-bellied pig as a pet and wondered if it should be castrated. In my answers to all of these, I tried to combine information with a sprinkling of humour, which can make such a difference on live television. The final caller, a lady from down south, had a dog with a very personal problem.

'Go on,' encouraged Richard, 'you can tell us.' He said this in a most persuasive way. The lady, thus coaxed to continue, told all to the audience of millions.

'Well, I'd like John to give me some help with my dog because he keeps making such embarrassing noises.' On the line we could just hear one of the 'noises' in the background. Judy looked slightly apprehensive, perhaps with some concern as to whether or not we should proceed with this line of questioning.

Quick as a flash, Richard was on to it. 'Was that your dog making a noise just now?' he asked.

'And what end of the dog was it coming from?' I chipped in, eager for clues.

The lady, now fully involved and quite enjoying her new-found notoriety, answered both of us simultaneously. 'That was a back-end one,' she said, 'but he does make noises from his front end as well.'

'Can you put him on?' asked Richard, and encouraged the caller to hold the phone down to the dog on the floor.

The dog 'performed' better than any of us expected, and that was the cue for chaos. Richard fell about, Judy rocked with uncontrollable laughter, despite the tone of the conversation. More importantly, the whole crew on the floor of the studio were audibly laughing through most of this episode.

'That's got to be a first,' said Richard, wiping the tears from his eyes, as the periodic reports still resounded from the phone. 'A farting dog on television!'

Of course, I made a vain attempt to give the lady a little more help amid all this enjoyable frivolity, but the farting dog on the phone was the real star, and even got Richard into the national press the very next day for being so rude on the telly.

As an associated follow-up to this flatulence episode, I decided next day to ring the lady with the pot-bellied pig, because I had promised some more detailed information that would not have been relevant during a live television programme. In the course of an interesting conversation, it did come out that these most wonderful pets did have one serious drawback. Being herbivorous animals, they apparently pass a lot of wind, and this tends to be a bit off-putting for visiting friends, who are unaware of the frequency of this behaviour, and the pungency of the odour! I sympathized with the lady's dilemma and explained that humans on high-fibre diets have the same problem.

'Ah yes,' she eagerly agreed, 'I know that, because I am also a vegetarian and I tend to have excessive flatulence. But,' she added, as I mused at what personal confidences people with common interests will divulge to each other, 'we can hold back a bit, can't we? We can wait to pass wind, until it is more appropriate, but a pig can't.'

Or won't, I thought, nodding silently at the phone.

'However,' she carried on a bit ruefully, 'I reckoned without the parrot.'

I snapped my brain back into wide-awake mode. 'Pardon?' I queried.

She explained. 'I used to wait until all my friends had gone, and then pass wind quite innocently in my own lounge.'

I imagined her vegetarian bowels relaxing into well-earned relief, as she 'let rip' in the privacy of her own home.

She then told me that the parrot, which also lived in the lounge and was an expert talker, picked up on these repeated performances and at her next dinner party, had its first mimicry try-out. As the excellent sound reproductions of a person passing wind echoed round the room, it was red faces all round. When moments later the source of the sound was traced to the parrot, then only one red face remained and it wasn't the bird's!

'What can I do?' she asked in all sincerity, as I fought not to burst out laughing on the phone. My mind, trained to instant response by years of live television, leaped into action.

'Blame it on the pig,' I said and put the phone down.

In my own small surgery set, the overall reaction of the crew is every bit as important as the multi-man set-up on the 'This Morning' set at Granada. Television is very much a team event and I am fortunate in having a superbly skilled group of technicians who are also human beings and happy to work together to produce programmes we can all be proud of!

On one occasion, I was set up to do a four-minute piece on exotic animals, and was standing behind my consulting-room table, with my animal stars concealed in a series of cardboard boxes. In my hands I held the biggest frog I have ever touched, and truly one of the most beautiful. He was, despite his brilliant green colour, called a White's tree frog, presumably after a man called White who first discovered him. It was much later he became a 'must' for television.

Like a great placid green lump, he sat calmly in my cupped hands, occasionally blinking his large baleful eyes, or silently swallowing with his balloon-like throat as if to let us know that he was still alive.

'Just take a look at this beautiful face,' I said directly to the camera, as Charlie zoomed in to fill the screen with the frog's magnificent green head. The frog turned slightly and offered Charlie a profile. After a bit of interesting banter on the frog's lifestyle and a close-up look at the suckers on the ends of its toes, I returned it to its box and recalled a recent programme where the great green frog had not been quite so well-behaved.

Because of the popularity of my own show, I was inevitably asked to contribute to others, and the opposition to ITV's 'This Morning', at that time was BBC's programme called 'Good Morning UK'. For the programme I was on, a young man called Adrian Mills was one of the presenters. As is often the case, producers like to use the universal appeal of animals to hook the viewers for the show ahead. So there I was, seated on the couch with the very same big green tree frog in my hands and Adrian was busy introducing the promise of the programme to come.

'As you may have already noticed, we have TV vet John Baxter here,' he said, 'who will be telling us some fascinating facts about the animals he has brought along, later in the programme.' All of his words rolled under the camera on his autocue, as he professionally delivered them word perfectly. As he finished, the next few seconds, although not scripted, made much better television. The green frog, who up to now, had been the perfect guest, looking good and not causing trouble, blotted his copy book. Whether he just got fed up or for some other froggy reason, he made one almighty jump and landed a good three feet away right on the young presenter's crotch. Adrian's face was a picture. As he hesitated, unsure of how to get this great frog off this very private part of his person, there was plenty of time for the cameras to pick up, not only his emotive expressions, but the cause of them, nestling on his nether regions.

Later, that same presenter moved on to the 'That's Life' team, and the clip of his embarrassingly good performance was used in the opening titles for the programme.

Back in my own surgery, I got on with my exotic theme.

'In here,' I said, in a more serious tone, 'are a couple of creatures which are not so cuddly.' Opening the box, I inclined my ear towards it. 'Listen,' I glanced towards the camera, as a loud hissing noise issued from the top of the open box. Well, that's what should have happened, but in actual fact, the expected hissing never materialized. I knew, however, that Charlie could sort that out later, so I professionally ploughed on. 'Never stop,' one old television hand once told me. 'unless the director tells you to.'

'These,' I said, lowering my voice to heighten the air of expectancy, 'these are hissing cockroaches from Madagascar.' So saying, I picked up one of the pair, which was about two-and-a-half inches long and half an inch wide, and placed it on the palm of my other hand. As it scampered, waving its inch-long antennae, it now needed no encouragement to hiss its disapproval at being disturbed. Grabbing it by the back of its mahogany-brown shell before it could take off up my arm, I continued. 'Don't be tempted,' I said, 'to do this with ordinary cockroaches, because unlike these Madagascar ones, ordinary cockroaches can carry a lot of disease.' I know that it was unlikely that anyone would ever even try to pick up a cockroach, but knowing the power of the telly, I considered the warning worthwhile. To further discourage any viewers from handling such creatures, I then up-ended the giant cockroach and showed the underside to the camera for a closer look.

'This is the bit that really puts me off,' I said quite truthfully, 'the "machinery" underneath.' As I did so, the cockroach pedalled its clawed legs and champed its mouth parts to emphasize my point. Bobbing it back with its mate, I closed the lid and wondered at the diversity of animal life in all its infinite variety.

Hissing cockroaches are not all that common, but I heard by chance that a school near Cambridge had some in their animal house, so I wrote asking them if they could let me have a pair for use on the telly. Around this same time, some of my nursing staff had noticed an entry in the personal column of the local newspaper professing a Miss Piggy's love for a Mr B. Unfortunately, Mr B was the abbreviated term that my staff used when speaking to me, so I had to take a bit of ribbing about who Miss Piggy was, and no amount of disclaimers appeared to allay their suspicions. So, when a small parcel arrived for Mr B's personal attention, hot on the heels of this newspaper nuisance, the girls were convinced that it was some kind of love token from Miss Piggy to me. As they gently shook the package at their ears in turn, in an attempt to ascertain the contents, I decided not to inform them that my diagnostic mind had already spotted the Cambridge postmark.

'Okay,' I said, 'if you are all so suspicious, you can open the parcel and satisfy yourselves of my innocence.'

There was no need for a second bidding as they set to with scissors and fingers to determine its romantic contents. If the impact on the viewers was even a quarter of the impact on my nurses when their eyes first saw the two giant cockroaches, then it would be dramatic indeed. With screams that all but drowned out the cockroaches' hissing, the two nurses leaped back a good three feet before fleeing from the room! Needless to say, Miss Piggy was never mentioned again.

The third of my little trio of unusual animals was as yet unseen by the crew. My visit to the Harewood Bird Gardens and my meeting with its curator had been more fruitful than they knew. I had only intended to borrow a tree frog, but after a quick scout through all the inmates, the curator confided in me that he had just received some rather special exhibits that very week. As its name suggests, Harewood Bird Garden is rightly famed for a spectacular collection of bird species, but it also has a section devoted to more terrestrial animals. As I followed the curator into the animal house, I could tell that he was as excited as I was.

'There are only another couple of these in the country,' he told me proudly, 'and they are at Edinburgh Zoo.'

'What exactly are they?' I asked, anxious to know at least roughly what to expect.

'Tomato frogs,' he replied without batting an eyelid. 'Have you ever seen any?'

Now equipped with the knowledge, not only of their rarity, but that the only other two in the country were in Scotland, I didn't hesitate to reveal my ignorance.

'No,' I replied. 'I've never even heard of them.' I mean, tomato frogs sounds more like the start for a music hall joke than the source of scientific inquiry.

'No,' said the curator, 'I'm not surprised. They are very shy.' Now my curiosity really was aroused! Tomato frogs and shy into the bargain! When in doubt always ask a question, my old professor at Glasgow Veterinary School had told me, so I launched my next query.

'Why do they call them tomato frogs then?'

The curator looked at me and laughed. 'Because they look like tomatoes,' he said, then switching to a more serious expression, he lifted down a plastic box about a foot square and six inches deep. 'They are in here,' he said, as we both peered cautiously down at the perforated lid.

'Remember,' he said, gently prising off the lid at one corner. 'They are very shy, so don't frighten them.'

Since this had never been my intention anyway, I nodded my agreement willingly. I don't quite know what I expected to see when he finally removed the lid completely, but certainly my first feelings were ones of disappointment. Nothing remotely like tomatoes, far less shy tomatoes, met my expectant gaze.

Instead, a large square of rotted turf lay facing me in the box. The curator looked at me out of the corner of his eyes and, seeing my look of disillusioned disbelief, he quickly added, 'They are so shy that they like to hide themselves away under decaying vegetation like this.' As he spoke he carefully turned back the turf to reveal two brilliantly red frogs, slightly cringing at the sudden exposure of their hiding place. I was amazed! They did look like tomatoes, they were timid, and they had that added ingredient which made them a must for any television programme. They were rare!

The curator kindly agreed to let me borrow them, along with the big green tree frog, and with a promise to look after them all with my life, I set out for the surgery with my precious charges.

Now, in the last box in the centre of the consulting-room table, I was ready for the exciting finale of this unusual animal piece.

'In this wee box,' I said, dramatizing all the stuff the curator had so recently taught me, 'are two of the rarest and the shyest frogs in the UK.' What I didn't tell the viewing audience was that I had the entire crew except for the cameraman standing in a semicircle around the table, just out of shot. 'This last animal,' I had told them, 'is very rare and very valuable. Trust me, it won't harm you. But,' I continued, putting on my most serious face, 'if by some unlucky chance it jumps from my hands, I want one of you to catch it. It is that rare and that valuable.'

With the crew like so many cricketing slip fielders, I felt the curator would have been proud of my care for his most rare and recent acquisitions. 'These,' I said, 'are tomato frogs, seen for the first time on British television.' I turned back the turf and Charlie moved in for a big close-up of the two timid frogs, now exposed to millions by the unexpected intervention of modern technology.

I picked up one of the plump red frogs and placed it on the palm of my extended left hand. In this position, I knew Charlie would get a good shot of the whole frog for all to see. What I didn't appreciate was that tomato frogs, like most of their other amphibian friends, are capable of leaping out of potentially hazardous situations at great speed. Neither had I noticed, in my attempt to rivet my TV audience, that my slip field of crew members were also so intrigued that their arms had dropped by their sides and their mouths hung slightly ajar in amazed disbelief at these strange creatures. Thus, they were in no ready state to anticipate far less catch the tomato frog, which leaped from my hand and, creating a spectacular arched flight path between the sound man and the producer, landed splat on the hard floor of the consulting room.

I hadn't the heart to tell the curator of the Bird Garden how close one of his new-found celebrities had come to being concussed, but I am sure that my secret was safe, because the tomato frog concerned was far too shy to talk about it anyway.

Chapter 11

Fishy Tales

'So Eric hasn't been eating properly for over two years?' I asked sympathetically.

'No,' Eric's owner replied, 'he just comes up to the surface, and we pop pieces of shrimp into his mouth, using a pair of chopsticks.'

A chance listener overhearing this conversation could be forgiven for wondering what we were talking about. But, for me, as a vet and a TV presenter, it was not only necessary to get a grasp of the facts but also to put Eric's owner at ease, before discussing his pet's problem in front of the cameras.

Being on television is for most people a nerve-wracking experience and few ever learn to be totally relaxed. For those who appear regularly on the screen as interviewers, the first priority should be to explain the ground rules and put the 'occasional performer' at his or her ease. Simply telling someone about to be interviewed to avoid looking directly at the camera and to ignore the crew is the least we can do. Some interviewers, of course, are so nervous themselves that they have little time or inclination to console anyone else. Fortunately, Eric's owner was a naturally unflappable type and, of course, Eric himself was blissfully unaware of what was about to happen.

Eric was a dog-faced puffer fish, who as you may have already gathered had an eating problem. His front teeth, which looked remarkably like human ones, had become so overgrown that they now wedged his mouth open and made it impossible for him to close his jaws.

Puffer fish, as their name suggests, can inflate their bodies when under threat. This makes them look more like footballs than fish. Such a rapid increase in volume no doubt frightens off any would-

A goldfish patient with a growth on the top of its head made a lasting impression when I gave a lecture on cryosurgery to surgeons in Florida.

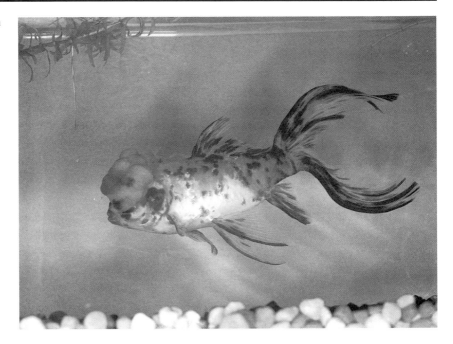

be attacker because, in Nature, big things are better left unmolested. An unfortunate side-effect of this defence strategy is that some inflated puffer fish get washed up on the shore and stranded like so many beach balls!

Some species of puffer fish, of which Eric was one, survive in the wild by nibbling fragments from the living coral and, as you will appreciate, this is a very hard material and it naturally keeps the fish's teeth well filed down. In captivity, with no such natural food source available, Eric's teeth had overgrown to leave him with his current problem.

Fish, I may say, form only a minute part of my patient list and anything I know about them has been gleaned from books, or from other fish experts I have met previously on filming locations.

One such visit to the Centre of Aquaculture at Stirling University introduced me to a brilliant professor who taught me more about these aquatic creatures in two hours than I had previously learned in my last ten years as a vet. One of the things I learned was how to anaesthetize fish, and having taught me this, the professor then offered me the opportunity to see the technique used in practice. That very day one of his young colleagues had to visit a salmon farm in a sea loch in the heart of the Scottish Highlands, and the crew was invited to join him. I drove in front with expert fish vet Hamish, and the crew followed on behind, in the television wagon with all the gear.

As we travelled through the spectacular Scottish countryside, Hamish regaled me with tales of the salmon industry and the threat put upon it by foreign producers. As vets always do, we talked 'shop' for the whole journey and only when we reached the sea loch did the breath-taking view stun us both into silence.

In the distance, I could see the circle of retaining tanks that housed the salmon in the middle of the loch and, beyond that, the blue heather-covered hills. Feeling every inch a Scotsman and now even a little bit like a fish vet, I followed Hamish's lead and donned some waterproof clothing and wellies. When the crew were likewise attired against the elements, we all headed out in a small boat, towards the fish farm. As a vet, I was thrilled by all the new knowledge I was acquiring and as a TV presenter, eager to find out more about Hamish's 'fishy' career.

Charlie, the director/cameraman and fellow Scot, was just as enthusiastic but his efforts were channelled in a different way. He had taken shots of Hamish and me leaving in the boat and then he had to clamber on to the platform that ran between the circular cages to take a shot of us arriving at the scene. Then there was the establishing shots to show where the farm fitted in to the general Highland scene and, of course, all the wee extra bits that Charlie was so expert at pulling out of his own broad experience. However, even Mike Best, the producer, was a bit doubtful when Charlie

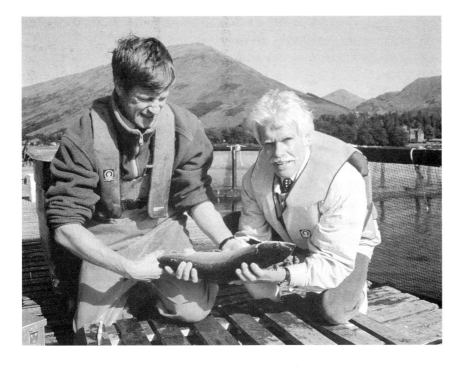

Fish vet, Hamish Rogers is an expert with Scottish salmon but as I was soon to find out, they could be very slippery customers.

donned a wet-suit and took an underwater camera into one of the salmon cages!

'It might only make ten seconds on the screen,' said Charlie, 'but it will really show the salmon's point of view and add depth to the whole piece.'

With that achieved, we had some first-class footage, but we still hadn't shot Hamish in action taking a blood sample from some of the three-foot-long salmon!

'Pass me that net, John,' said Hamish, anxious to get on and, taking it from me, he leaned over the wall of the cage and scooped out a couple of beautiful fish. Another scoop and two more joined their mates in a holding tank on the ramp.

'If you want to help,' said Hamish, appreciating my eagerness to be involved, 'you can transfer one of the fish into the anaesthetic tank.' He nodded towards a second blue fibreglass tank, into which he had previously poured an anaesthetic drug.

Deftly in with the net again, and Hamish and I had moved one of the salmon over, gently rolling it from the folds of the netting into the second tank.

'How long should it take, Hamish?' I asked, keen to know every detail of a technique which I could use back in my surgery.

'Och, about two minutes at the most,' Hamish replied, and as he spoke the large fish started to become disorientated, then rolled over on one side and hung quite limp in the water. 'Okay John. Lift it out onto this board for me,' Hamish instructed, as he got his syringe and needle ready for the blood sampling.

On camera or not, this was my big moment, and as I gently lifted the sedated salmon out of the anaesthetic tank I could appreciate not only how heavy it was, but also how very slippery! The fish had scarcely been put down before Hamish was delicately probing at its rear end to draw blood from a vein he couldn't even see! As the bright red blood pulled back into the syringe, he explained that by screening for a whole series of substances in the blood he could help prevent disease processes before they got started.

'Good,' he said, obviously pleased with his efforts. I knew just how relieved he must have felt. It's all very well doing your everyday work efficiently but, believe me, it is ten times harder when a television camera is watching your every move. 'Now you can pop it back with the rest of the salmon in the main tank before it comes round too far.'

Like Hamish, my veterinary-trained eyes had also noted the increased gill movements and we both knew that the fish was 'getting light' and starting to revive as the anaesthetic wore off.

That's when disaster so nearly struck! Whether it was the imminent recovery of the fish, its slippery scales or perhaps some slight movement it made, I will never know. I had it precariously supported in both my hands and when I extended my arms to lift it over the barrier and back into the tank, it slipped from my grasp and fell, not into the cage, but into the loch itself.

'Hamish, help!' I cried out, seeing my loss of a prime salmon hitting some Scottish newspaper headlines!

'Conservation-mad TV vet throws three-foot salmon back into loch!' The reporters would have a field day.

Hamish, who was getting set up for blood sampling the next salmon, leaped to his feet and with a speed I would have thought impossible in wellies, dashed to my side. He dipped his arms deep into the water of the loch and grabbed the still half-dopey salmon by its tail. Gently but firmly, he pulled it to the surface and expertly transferred it back into the tank. Being a kind-hearted person, Hamish did not make as much fuss about my mistake as the crew did. Nevertheless, I did manage to have the last laugh by boasting to my friends back home about the majestic salmon I had caught in the Highlands, and then so nearly lost again!

I was surprised that I had spent such a pleasurable day on the Scottish loch because, to be honest, I have always had quite an aversion to water. I have tended to subscribe to Billy Connolly's philosophy that the human species took millions of years to climb out of the sea, so why should we ever want to plunge back into it!

If I ever needed reminding of that sobering thought, I got my most punishing lesson whilst fishing at Portpatrick off the west coast of Scotland.

Charlie the director had decided that the stuff we shot at Deep Sea World in North Queensferry was pretty good, but lacked that little something to make it sparkle.

In the course of filming this aquatic exhibition, it had come to light that all the fish in 'the largest freshwater tank in the world' had been caught in the offshore waters around the British Isles. Even more surprisingly, they had not been netted but caught with a rod and line. Currently, the two intrepid anglers who supplied the fish were based at Portpatrick, so with the bit now firmly between his teeth, Charlie led us off to see for ourselves.

When we arrived at this tiny picturesque fishing village, it was late evening and the coloured lights around the harbour gave the whole scene a fairy-like quality. Full of optimism, we booked into a local hotel and looked forward to joining the fishermen on the following morning as they set out into the Atlantic in search of fish.

Next morning Portpatrick didn't look quite so pleasing. Rain drizzled down and the sea looked distinctly choppy. Undaunted by this, Charlie sheltered under a multicoloured umbrella and with Ian the sound man by his side, started to film the loading of a large shark. This fish was being put into a tank on the lorry waiting at the quayside and Charlie continued to film it as it made its way along Portpatrick's main street and then on southwards to North Queensferry.

With the ending of the piece in the 'can', now all we had to do was film the trip to sea and hopefully catch another fish which would double for the one already heading for Deep Sea World.

From the moment I clambered aboard that very small boat and cheerily greeted the two weather-beaten fishermen I had a premonition of trouble ahead. As I began collecting some background details from the young Australian skipper, my stomach started sending messages to my brain that all was not well!

The bottom of the tiny craft slapped into bigger and bigger waves as it headed further out to sea. I frantically tried to keep my eyes on the distant horizon as feelings of nausea rose in my stomach. I glanced back at the receding coastline with Portpatrick just visible through the sea spray and prayed I would be able to do my bit without vomiting.

'Right John,' said Charlie, with an enviable enthusiasm in his voice, 'I'll get them to cut the engines and stop the boat and then you can do the main interview with the captain.'

'Cut the engines and stop the boat.' The words fell on my ears with the promise of salvation. I convinced myself that I would be alright when the boat stopped. How wrong I was!

The engines cut and sure enough the boat stopped going out to sea, but it was far from motionless. If anything, it rocked about on the spot with increased momentum. Charlie called for 'Action' and the Aussie cast his line out to sea and then turned to me. Whether his look of mild surprise was due to nerves at being filmed for telly or provoked by the rapidly changing colour of my complexion I will never know. Neither will I know how I got through that interview, and to be honest, I could care even less. I only know that it was not the lack of questions which brought the discussion to an abrupt halt but more my need to reach over the side and vomit repeatedly.

As I watched my hotel breakfast disperse in the agitated waters of the Atlantic, I wondered if this TV caper was really worth all the effort.

Back on dry land and feeling well enough to try a pub lunch, I was naturally the object of the whole community's jokes. What I didn't realize until later was that the sound recordist had also gone green at the gills and even managed to be sick over the side whilst I was doing that fateful interview.

'But,' said Charlie, ever the purist, 'if you had been well enough, John, you would have noticed that although he vomited over the side, the position of the boom mike he was holding for your interview never budged! That's the mark,' he added jokingly, 'of a true professional.'

'Well, tell me this, Charlie,' I was now feeling quite good-natured, what with being back on terra firma and having a half of lager in my hand, 'how come you never felt queasy?'

Charlie's retort was instant. 'Ah well, you see, John. I just keep my eye on the camera viewfinder and pretend I'm watching television.'

Now, in the familiar surroundings of my own surgery, where the operating theatre was doubling as a studio set, I looked down into Eric's tank and weighed up the task ahead. I had taken the precaution

Aquatic expert, Howard Tolliday, and I get into wet suits to talk about some fishy inmates at Deep Sea World in Scotland.

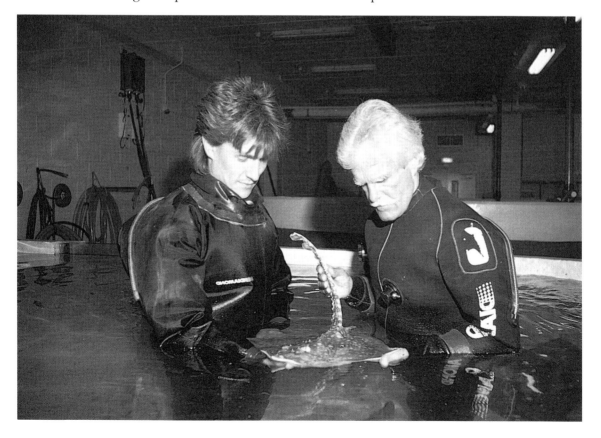

of calling in a local aquarist to assist me in the operation and equipped with my new-found knowledge on fish anaesthesia, I had a separate tank all prepared. Eric's owner netted his pet fish with a dexterity derived from his daily feeding routine and carefully transferred him into the anaesthetic tank.

Two and a half minutes later, Eric, unstressed and still his normal size, lay sleeping on a moistened foam pad on my operating table. Knowing that he would be quite safe for a few minutes, I grabbed my dental drill, fitted it with a special diamond saw wheel, and started to trim back his overgrown teeth. Cutting the teeth, formed as they were of solid enamel, proved no easy task, but when I had finished, Eric's still-sleeping mouth could be closed to perfection.

'Pop him back in his own tank now,' I urged his owner, who had been standing anxiously by watching the whole procedure with an air of disbelief.

Eric plopped, limp, into his home tank and slowly wafted down to the bottom.

'Will he be all right?' I heard his owner nervously ask over my shoulder as we all peered into the tank. I waited a moment until Eric's gill and fin movement increased so that I could add confidence to my reply.

'Sure, he'll be fully round in a few minutes,' I said.

True to my forecast, Eric's face brightened up, his fins went into action and he was soon swimming around his tank completely unaware of the saga in which he had been the main player.

'Drop in a piece of shrimp,' I instructed the now delighted owner, 'and let's see what he will do.'

Smiling all over his face, Eric's owner did just that and the fish immediately grabbed the piece of shrimp and gobbled it down. If we had had a studio audience, I have little doubt that they would have burst into spontaneous applause, not because we had filmed my first bit of puffer fish dentistry, but because veterinary science had allowed a little fish to eat his first meal for two years, under his own steam.

All I could say was, 'Well done Eric!'

Chapter 12

Foreign Locations

One of the many things I like about making television programmes featuring my own profession is the opportunity I get to watch other vets in action.

As with any other group of 'workers' there are those who stand out in my memory as being extra-special and one such vet went under the splendid name of Doctor Kuno von Plocki!

As the series of 'It's a Vet's Life' gained in popularity and moved from being a local series on Yorkshire Television to going national on the ITV network, things changed. Because of the competition for network slots and a bigger budget, we were no longer limited to Yorkshire or even the UK when it came to selecting film locations. I still elected to keep the same small crew, but in order to give the national series a bit of added quality we set off for some European locations. We loaded up a Ford Transit van with all our gear, and travelled to France, Belgium, Holland and Germany to seek out suitable stories for the eight programmes of the series.

The first stop was Paris, and the famous Pasteur Institute, where Louis Pasteur, 'the father of medicine', did all his wonderful work on rabies and vaccine production.

I know there must be many of you who enjoy viewing great works of art, listening to classical music or visiting the houses of the rich and famous. For me, none of these can hold a candle to walking on the hallowed ground of the Pasteur Institute. Nothing could have impressed me more than sitting in that little room, at the very desk where the great Pasteur must have agonized over his innovative theories and been overjoyed when they proved correct.

'Vill you just let your arm relax, John,' said the delightful German lady doctor. 'You von't feel a thing!' I smiled at the camera as Doctor

Louis Pasteur was rightly called the father of medicine and it was a wonderful experience to sit at the very desk where he did so much of his pioneering work.

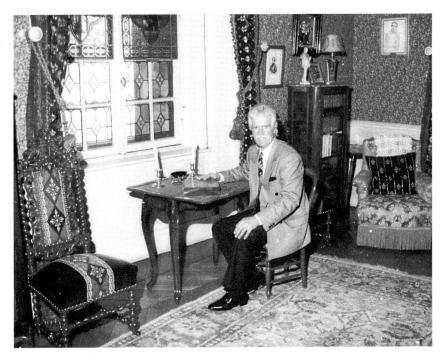

Monika Hertzog administered the first part of my vaccination against rabies and I marvelled at how far rabies research had progressed. Gone were the painful injections into the stomach, now it was a simple jab in the arm like many other vaccines.

In Pasteur's day rabies was a real killer for which there was no known treatment. Anyone bitten by a rabid 'mad dog' was certain to die. Pasteur developed a vaccine from infected rabbits' spinal cords and with this, he was instrumental in saving many people infected with the rabies virus. Perhaps his most spectacular success involved a young boy called Joseph Meister, who had been bitten by a mad dog and was the first person to be saved by the revolutionary new rabies vaccine. Joseph not only survived, but grew up to become the doorman at the famous Institute where the life-saving vaccine had been produced. Sad to say, in 1940 when the invading German army entered Paris, a loyal Joseph Meister had tried to prevent some soldiers from entering a chapel which had been erected in Pasteur's memory, and for his efforts was shot dead.

'Okay John, you can roll down your sleeve now,' said the doctor. I smiled and gave her a kiss on the cheek. I knew it would look good on camera! 'Zank you for being so kind,' she said, 'and as for all my brave little patients, I give you this.' She opened the drawer of her desk and gave me a sweet!

That episode in Monika's rabies clinic made a nice little interview about a very serious subject, but not one hundred yards away, in another part of the Institute there was something a bit more grisly going on.

Every day sacks arrive at the gatekeeper's lodge containing boxes for scientific examination at the Institute. These boxes, we learned, contained the severed heads of dogs which had been destroyed because they were suspected of having rabies. The only conclusive proof of this possibility was to open up the skulls and directly examine the brain tissue for the rabies virus. Naturally, all of the technicians doing this skilled work were protected by vaccination. My film crew were not, and I had only just had my first shot.

As we stood outside the sealed room, I could see the gowned and masked technicians going about their gruesome work, and as I

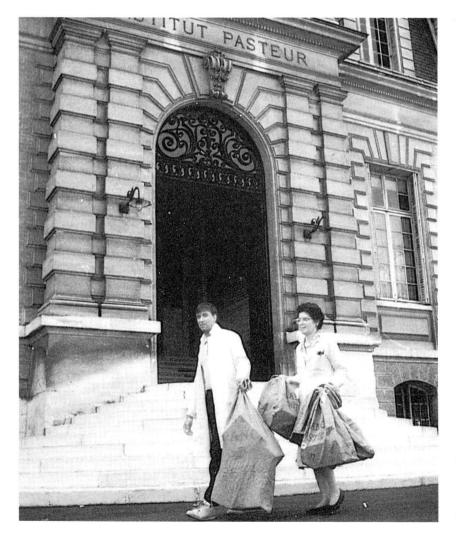

Medical technicians at the Pasteur Institute collect sacks containing the severed heads of dogs which are to be used for rabies testing.

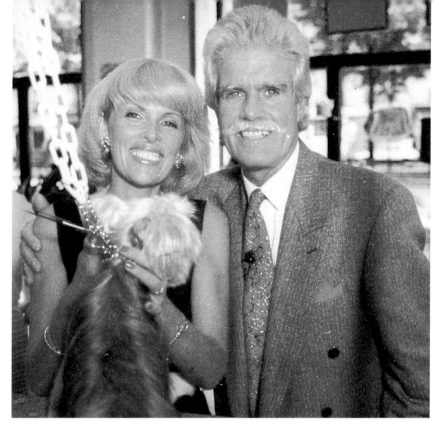

The glamorous owner of a poodle parlour in Paris gives me a demonstration in canine coiffeur – French style.

talked to the camera about the lethal rabies virus which was just behind the glass, I could feel the hair rise on the back of my neck.

Rabies is still very much a threat in Europe and elsewhere and although Pasteur's work has helped save many human lives, there is still much to be done in eradicating the disease from wild life.

Thank goodness we don't have rabies in Great Britain!

As if by contrast, our next stop was at a Parisian poodle parlour to see the flamboyance and the wonderfully extravagant style of some pet owners in this capital city. It was an intentionally flippant piece and it did help raise our spirits after dealing with the grim subject of rabies. Then, it was back into the Transit, and a long drive to our hotel in Holland, so that we could make an early start in the morning to meet a lady who had devoted her whole life to seals.

The seal sanctuary was in a small town called Pieterburen. The lady in charge, whose name was at first unpronounceable, was called Lenie t' Hart. However, any difficulties I might have had with her name, were more than made up for by her generously warm personality and her deep-felt dedication to her beloved 'Zeehunden'.

Through plate-glass viewing panels, we watched some blubber-fat young seals sleeping underwater and I saw the joy on Lenie's face, as she explained every detail of their behaviour to me.

'They are mammals just like us, John,' she said. 'And although they can stay under water for much longer than we can, they still have to come to the surface to breathe, just occasionally. There, see!' She pointed at one still fast-asleep youngster, who like an over-inflated balloon, was just starting to float gently towards the surface. There, with his eyes still closed, he breathed in another full quota of oxygen and slowly drifted back down again, with his eyes still closed.

'Watch, watch,' said Lenie, with a girlish enthusiasm, as the young seal 'touched down' on the bottom of the pool. We both laughed quite genuinely as the little over-blown seal bounced like a rubber ball until he came to rest and settled once more into the peaceful stillness of deep sleep.

On a more serious note, Lenie showed us her isolation units where young seals in varying degrees of illness were being helped back to health.

'That one there,' she pointed through the glass, 'is suffering from a dreadful distemper-like virus. Terrible,' she said, shaking her head, and I could tell that the disease which had killed so many seals had also caused Lenie many hours of sadness.

Before I could dwell too long on that depressing illness, I was reminded by Lenie that caring for sick animals was very much my

Charlie Flynn, the cameraman/director of 'It's a Vet's Life' films me and seal nurse, Anita giving some tender loving care to one of the seal patients at the Sanctuary.

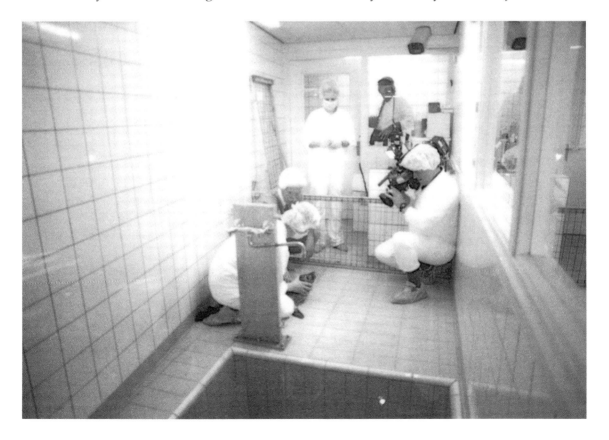

own role in life. So, dressed in a sterile white suit, with matching wellies, I found myself inside the quarantine room, and helping a charming seal nurse called Anita to force feed one of the ailing youngsters. As she skilfully straddled the patient on the floor and passed a rubber tube into its stomach, I connected a plastic funnel onto the other end and tipped in a bellyful of mushed-up fish food.

Judging by the struggle that little chap put up and Anita's flushed cheeks, I reckoned that this was one little seal who was well on the way to recovery.

From Pieterburen we travelled to Germany and as the Transit headed into the pine-covered hills between Strasbourg and Stuttgart, both Charlie, an Aberdonian, and myself, a Fifer, were most impressed by the country's similarity to Scotland. The scenery was certainly spectacular and as we approached the Schwarzwald (the Black Forest), we came upon Doctor Kuno von Plocki's veterinary centre or Tierklinik.

Kuno could not have been more polite or more professionally accommodating. A man in his late forties or early fifties, he had a slim and well-exercised figure which went well with his handsome features. The merest hint of a foreign accent came through his impeccable English and gave an overall effect which I felt could make most middle-aged ladies swoon at fifty paces.

'What can I show you, John?' he asked politely, after I had formally introduced myself and the crew.

'I'd like to see everything you have got, Kuno,' I replied, eager to explore the premises of this successful equine vet, who not only served as the official veterinary surgeon for the German National Show-jumping team, but for the Olympic team as well.

Charlie the director and Mike the producer were always keen for me to take a preliminary look at each location and see what it might yield in the way of usable story lines, while they unloaded and sorted out the film gear. Afterwards I would relay to them the material I had found and they would use this as a basis for the filming schedule.

'This is my recovery ward,' said Kuno, unbolting the stable doors, and showing me a mare who was a recently recovered post-operative case. A row of stitches in her lower abdomen marked Kuno's surgical intervention to relieve a twist in her bowel.

'And what about these bandages on her front legs, Kuno?' I asked, not seeing the point of them at all.

'Well you see, John, when these horses come in with colic or other bowel problems, they are in such pain that they thrash their legs against the sides of the horse-box. Nearly all of them,' he added, 'injure themselves in this way.'

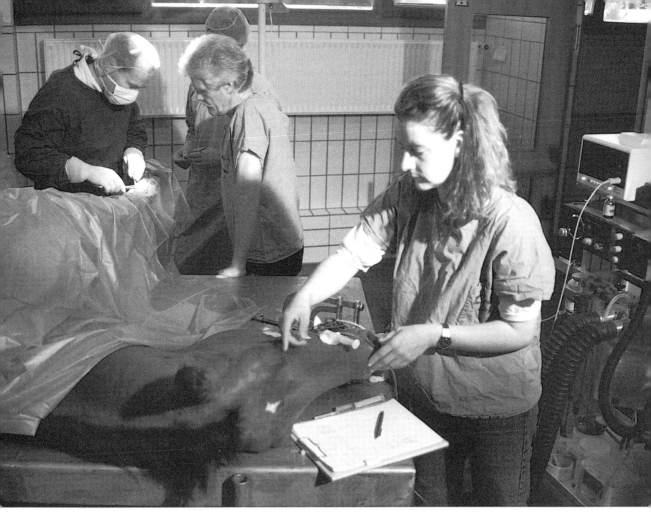

As we made our way along the ward, the fact that almost every horse had bandaged front legs was a testament to his explanation.

Over the years, Kuno has become a recognized expert in the field of emergency bowel surgery and because of this and his expertise in many other aspects of equine work, patients would be brought from as far away as Belgium and Switzerland to benefit from his skills.

Later that morning, I had a chance to see him in action as he calmly anaesthetized a thoroughbred and skilfully corrected a tendon abnormality in its foreleg. While we were recording that operation on film, I asked Kuno if he had ever come across rabies, as I knew it existed in that area from my visit to the Pasteur Institute.

'Rabies? Rabies?' Kuno looked up from the operation with a bewildered expression on his face. 'What is rabies?'

I looked at him in disbelief. Here was a highly respected and intelligent vet and he didn't know what rabies was!

'La Rage,' I offered the French version and that did the trick.

'Ah!' his face lit up with the realization of what I was talking about. 'You mean Tollvut.'

In his clinic on the edge of the Black Forest, an exceptional German horse vet shows me some of the finer points of equine surgery.

Now, it was my turn to be humble. Of course, the German for rabies is Tollvut.

'Ja! Ja!' I relaxed into the little bit of German I knew! *'Enschuldigen Sie bitte*. Excuse me!'

Kuno then told me of a recent real-life tale, which was every bit as chilling to me as the dissections of the brains at the Pasteur Institute.

With the slightest increase in his German accent, probably brought on by the recall of his story, he related the sequence of events to me.

'As you now know, my friend, I am almost totally absorbed with the medicine and surgery of horses, and I very seldom come into contact with dogs, cats and the like.' He looked down at the operation site to check that all was well, and continued. 'Sometimes, however, the local vet will ask me to help on some matter or other, and about a year ago now, he was having trouble catching a client's dog which had gone a bit wild. He wondered if I could give him a hand. I took some stout gloves and set off into the village to confront the dog. When I got there I found that the animal was very aggressive and whenever anyone approached, it would growl viciously.' He swallowed anxiously and went on. 'Just when I thought I had it round the throat with my gloved hands, it slipped free and bit me on the face!' Kuno went visibly pale at the recollection of his ordeal and I already guessed what he was about to tell me.

'And the dog had rabies, Tollvut?' I asked.

'The dog died and a post mortem was done which confirmed that it had Tollvut,' he repeated solemnly. 'I can tell you, John,' he said with conviction, 'I have never been so terrified in all my life. And you will know, that the closer you are bitten to your brain, the faster you develop the disease. I had been bitten on the face!' He licked his lips and went on. 'Of course I had the vaccine straight away, but I didn't sleep for the next five days because I knew that it was a life and death race between the vaccine and the rabies virus. If the virus won,' he said solemnly, 'I knew I would die.'

It was every vet's worst nightmare!

Kuno bent down again to suture the wound on the horse's leg and I mentally congratulated myself on having my first rabies shot at the Pasteur Institute.

Just as Kuno was placing the last stitch, as if on cue, the operating theatre door burst open, and a nurse shouted an urgent message which my school-level German failed to decipher.

Kuno was quick to translate and Charlie even quicker to respond.

'Apparently,' said Kuno, 'a horse-box has arrived with a mare who is down and is looking pretty bad.'

Whilst Kuno's staff took over the care of the patient on the operating table, we all dashed outside to help with the emergency.

The first thing we heard was the ominous noise of a horse in terrible pain, beating its hooves on the wooden walls of the box. In a small anxious knot, the owners of the horse and their relatives stood awaiting Kuno's help. One of the nurses and myself tried to push shut the side door of the box which had been forced open by a kick from the horse. As we did so, I caught sight of the shocked look of desperation on the mare's face as she lay fighting for her life. Even as a pet vet, I could tell that it would take more than Kuno's undoubted skill to save her.

I looked at Kuno's face as his nurse gave the horse a pain-killing shot in her buttock. I could see that he too knew that the mare was already beyond help. After a few sympathetic words with the tearful group, he turned to me.

'It appears, John, that the mare is six months in foal and they have travelled over two hundred kilometres to get here.' He shook his head sadly. 'If only I could have got at it two hours sooner, I know that I could have saved her.'

As he spoke, I saw the mare give a long sigh and the thrashing and the noise suddenly ceased.

'Is there no chance of at least saving the foal, Kuno?' I asked in the vain hope that a Caesarean section on the dead mare might give her unborn foal a chance of life.

'I am afraid not, John,' said Kuno sadly, 'at six months old it would have no chance of survival.'

All that was left no was the grieving of the horse's owners and a long sad journey home with an empty horse-box.

After this dramatic episode, all we had to do was to shoot a final interview with Kuno. As we sat in his office and discussed how horses had become the love and purpose of his whole life, I could see the tiredness that overwork and stress can bring to a dedicated vet. We thanked him for his hospitality and set off down the winding road through the forest, pleased to have had such a successful day's filming but sad to have witnessed the final struggles of a brave horse.

At the bottom of the hill, against a scenic backdrop, Charlie decided that here, next to the main road, would be a good place for me to do 'an opening piece to camera'. Back at base this would then be edited in to make the opening introduction to our film with Kuno.

Trouble came twofold with this idea. First we had to wait until there was a gap in the fast-moving traffic and, second, I had to be word-perfect with a script which could have tripped up the most eloquent of presenters. It went something like this.

'Today we have come to a very special veterinary centre, a Tierklinik on the edge of the Schwarzvald or Black Forest to meet an exceptional horse vet called Doctor Kuno von Plocki, who might realistically be described as the Harley Street consultant of the horse world.'

Between the cars and my verbal slip-ups, it took ten attempts to get it right. In the end, the producer was delighted. I was overjoyed at finally triumphing against such colossal odds and even Ian the sound man, never one to be readily impressed, thought the quality was okay. Unfortunately Charlie the director decided it didn't quite fit, and after all my efforts, dropped it!

Chapter 13

Swan Song

I kept perfectly still and quiet, as the lady vet made the last few delicate incisions through the muscles that had once given the patient such power of movement.

At times like this the viewing public could sense the tension and glib talk was the last thing they would want to hear. I could see out of the corner of my eye that Charlie was tight on a shot of the lady vet's hands cutting away, but as soon as the white bone of the limb came into view, he pulled back to a wider shot. It wasn't too upsetting for Charlie, but he had quite rightly decided that it might be too much for the viewing public to handle.

'So the next step is to sever the bone of the wing?' I asked the young vet an obvious question, by way of explaining the situation to a future audience.

With patches of sweat appearing through her green operating gown, as she approached the end of the op, she nodded her agreement and replied, 'Yes John, and if you would like to pass me the bone saw I'll get it done.' Her voice was a bit muffled and distant through her surgical mask and I could see by Ian's expression that he was not too happy with the sound quality. Mind you, that was nothing unusual for Ian. A perfectionist by nature, he was never one hundred per cent satisfied with anything that passed through his earphones. He was always striving for a better mike position, less extraneous interference or, simply, a bit more precise speech from presenters like myself. All of these things he demanded, but in such a pleasant way and with such a non-critical air, that it was impossible to be upset by his requests. Ian was a nice man with a high degree of technical skill and everyone wanted for him what he wanted for himself.

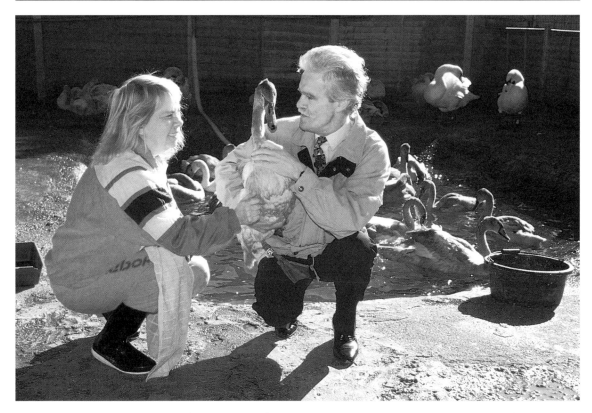

Swans are magnificent and graceful birds – they could not have a more devoted fan than Dot Beeson MBE.

The noise of the saw cutting through the bone brought me back to reality and I looked down on the magnificent white swan that lay anaesthetized on the table. I wondered how she would cope with life after having her wing amputated.

This was my first time working with birds as big as swans. As a pet vet, it was, of course, a daily occurrence for me to deal with budgies and I did realize that the smallness of my patients brought hazards of its own. Diagnosis, for instance, sometimes had to be much more the result of educated guesswork, than the objective results of listening with a stethoscope or feeling with fingers, no matter how skilled and sensitive they might be.

In my early days as a vet, one lady owner had me stumped from the very beginning.

'My wee budgie,' she announced on the telephone, in an anxious voice, 'is not very well.' She hesitated, and I checked my watch. Eleven o'clock on a Sunday evening, I thought to myself. A fine time to notice that her budgie was not very well.

As if the pause had conveyed my lack of belief in the urgency of her budgie's condition, she continued with a little more stridency in her tone of voice, 'and...and he is sweating profusely!'

That did it. A budgie sweating profusely had to be seen. 'I'll be right over,' I said, 'and don't do anything until I get there.'

I meant, of course, that she should not attempt to do anything with the bird. I didn't want her trying to solve the budgie's problem with a hairdryer! As I climbed into my car and started the engine, my mind struggled with the possible causes of such a situation. Like most people faced with a difficult problem, I first tried to allot the blame elsewhere.

Five years at Glasgow Veterinary School, I said to myself with righteous indignation, and never a mention of sweating budgies!

When I reached the house, a frail lady in her late fifties answered the door and welcomed me in.

'Sorry to call you out so late, Doctor, but Billy's got me really worried.' Shuffling into her living room, hands clasped in front of her, she nodded her greying head towards the birdcage which stood in one corner of the room. 'That's him, Doctor. He doesn't look well, does he?'

One glance at Billy's bedraggled and sodden figure sitting dejectedly on the perch was enough to convince me that 'not looking well' had to be the medical understatement of the year.

Still clueless as to the cause of Billy's pitiful condition, I remained silent in the face of the owner's repeated description of her bird's condition. 'He is sweating pretty badly though, Doctor, isn't he?'

I walked silently towards the fireplace wracking my brains for any past reference to any disease remotely like Billy's problem. I even resorted to holding my folded stethoscope against my temple to imply to the distraught owner that I was indeed, a 'doctor' deep in deductive thought.

'...and,' she added, increasing the volume of her voice as if to redirect my observations back to Billy, 'he has a hole in his head!'

It worked a treat! In a trice, I was back by the cage and peering at the hole in Billy's head. At least, now, part of my education seemed to be paying off. The hole in the bird's head was quite natural. It was his ear-hole! Normally concealed by the bird's plumage, only the parting of the bird's sodden feathers had exposed it. My explanation of this fact seemed to rebuild a little of my reputation with Billy's owner.

Hot on the heels of my ear-hole success, I decided to resort to the vet's basic bottom-line technique. Observation! Animals can't talk, so look for objective signs of disease.

Billy was certainly soaking wet and as my newly confident medical approach blossomed, my eyes scanned his immediate environment for clues, and there they were! Telltale splashes of damp on the floor of his cage. The solution was obvious.

Billy wasn't sweating at all! He had merely slipped from his perch and nose-dived into his own water dish!

The big bird on the table in front of me was certainly no budgie, and her problem was very real indeed.

'Just put the wing over on the side, John,' directed the vet, now visibly relieved that the worst was over.

Although it was the first time I had ever been involved in the amputation of a swan's wing, I had had plenty of experience of limb amputations in dogs and cats. As I took the wing in my gloved hands, the feeling was all too familiar. In the seconds it took to lift it and discard it, I had a feeling of revulsion mixed with sadness. A few minutes previously, it had been attached as a vital and integral part of the living body of an animal. Now, with bone and muscle attachments severed and the blood and nerve supply cut, it still retained the form, but none of the function, of a wing. As always, it was a relief for me to get it out of my sight and concentrate my mind on the final stitching that would finish the job.

All of this was taking place at the Swan Sanctuary at Egham, where our crew and cameras had come to film the work of a very remarkable lady called Dot Beeson, who now stood quietly in one corner of the room as her vet put in the final sutures and dressed the wound. Dot is not one for hogging the limelight. She took her cue, though, when Charlie looked up from the camera eyepiece at the end of the op. While the vet left to get cleaned up, Dot scooped up the still unconscious swan and, holding the great bird close to her breast, carried it out of the operating theatre and into the recovery ward.

Away from the limelight of the filming scene, Dot was much more relaxed and as she showed me round the ward, her dedication to the welfare of these majestic birds was very evident. With her latest patient bedded down, she gave me a guided tour.

'These two here,' she said, pointing to a couple of poorly looking specimens, 'are just getting over lead poisoning. You will know, John,' she said, assuming that as a vet I would know more about swans than she did, 'that an awful lot of swans die from lead poisoning by swallowing anglers' lead weights. With a bit of luck though,' she added optimistically, 'we'll save these two. And that one over there,' she indicated a solitary swan with a bandage round its neck, 'is fine now. We're just waiting to remove his stitches, then he'll be off.'

'So what did you have to do for that one, Dot?' I asked, eager to pick up all I could on swan ailments.

'Oh, that one managed to swallow a bit of discarded fishing line and unfortunately, it still had a hook attached. Imagine,' she continued, showing her true concern for her patients, 'how much that poor bird must have suffered.'

Running her short fingers through her blonde hair, Dot dashed round the ward with boundless energy, giving me a completely new perspective on swan ailments and injuries. There were swans there which even Dot's optimistic approach couldn't hope to save but, as expected, she was determined that she would give them every comfort as long as they weren't in pain.

In the last pen was a beautiful female swan who appeared in the peak of health and vigour, except that she had, on closer inspection, a little bit of an unbalanced look.

'That's Dolly,' she said, with affection. 'She had a wing amputated four weeks ago, after she flew into a telegraph pole. Swans,' she further explained, 'are a bit accident-prone, and we are forever getting them in with wing injuries caused by them flying into man-made objects. That one the vet treated today, flew into a railway bridge, which unfortunately lies directly in line with the swans' flight path down to the lake.'

'And what happens to the swans that have their wings amputated, Dot?' I asked. 'Do they just become long-term, disabled inmates in your sanctuary?'

'No John, the great thing about swans,' she replied, 'is that they mate for life. If we keep them here in one of our ponds then other swans, flying over, may decide to drop in. If then, as often happens, a swan visitor pairs up with one of our amputees, we know that their love is for life. After a suitable bonding period, we can then release them to people who have large ponds or lakes on their land, and they can live happily ever after, swimming about and looking lovely in their new home. Actually,' said Dot, 'we are bringing in the male cob, who is the husband of the swan you saw in the ward today, so that you can see what I mean about this lifelong bond.'

The cob duly arrived with some of Dot's helpers later that afternoon, and with the aid of a long canvas carrier bag, we transported him to the pond where his mate was having her first swim around since losing her wing. Whilst the cameras recorded this happy event for all to see, Dot and I stood spellbound at the miracle of their reunion, and I could only admire and respect an ordinary lady who had done such extraordinary things for the birds that she loves.

Later, one of her helpers showed me the British Empire Medal which Dot had received for her work with swans, and allowed me to read a very special letter from the Queen, giving Dot Beeson the responsibility for looking after any injured swans on the 'Royal' river Thames.

One of the most important factors in making an interesting television series, is the finding of unusual and sometimes unique personalities to feature in the programmes. For me, Dot Beeson, MBE, was certainly one of them.

In my work, both as a vet and as a television presenter, I had had quite a lot of experience with birds that were most times sick, but sometimes just a bit too healthy!

On one location, I had the unenviable task of trying to interview the lady owner of a birds of prey centre. She was undoubtedly an expert in the training and handling of birds of prey, but her enthusiasm for her work sometimes bubbled over into an

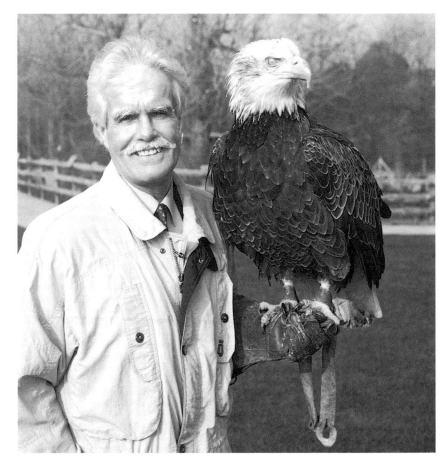

One of my most exhilarating experiences on 'It's a Vet's Life' came when a magnificent bald eagle swooped in from about 200 yards away and landed on my outstretched arm.

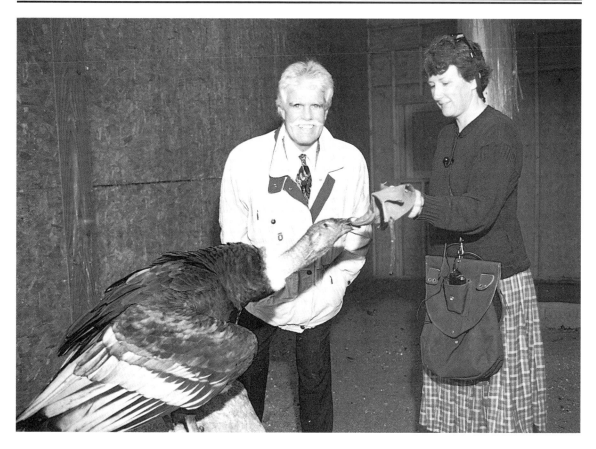

extroversion which was hard to contain. Like her father before her, who founded the centre, she was perfectly at home with all her avian inmates, and even the biggest and most threatening birds seemed to know that she respected and cared for them deeply.

Perhaps that's why the director thought it a pretty novel idea for me to interview her in the cage of a giant condor! For those who are unfamiliar with this species of bird, just make a mental picture of an immense vulture with a strong broad hooked beak some eight inches long.

'Come on John,' she said, dragging me into the great bird's den, and securing a large metal door behind us. 'We don't want our friend here to escape.'

I must admit that my route of escape was more important to me than any thought of the bird gaining its freedom! High above us, perched on a realistic rockface, the condor fixed us with a penetrating gaze. I noted that Charlie and the crew were filming through the bars of the cage in comparative safety. I looked at the bird lady and judged that she was a little too small for me to hide behind.

A hairy moment for any presenter as a 'killer' condor is kept at bay by an avian expert with her bag of tit-bits.

'Couldn't we start the interview and hope that he might fly overhead?' I suggested timidly through the bars to Charlie.

The bird lady answered the question before Charlie had time to open his mouth.

'Come on down, son,' she coaxed the great bird, digging her hand into a leather pouch which was slung over her shoulder. 'Come on, darling,' she repeated her invitation and held a piece of meat upwards in her outstretched hand by way of added incentive.

If I had, at that moment, been facing the camera, the expression of fear it would have recorded might well have damaged my reputation as a vet. Budgies and even parrots I could handle, but as this great condor swooped down to alight at my feet, I nearly fainted and joined it on the floor!

'Just make sure you keep me between yourself and the bird John,' cautioned the bird lady, for the first time confirming that there was real danger here. The condor tore the piece of meat from her grasp and gulped it down.

Transfixed by the awesome power of the bird's massive hooked beak, I heard, as though through a dream, Charlie's call for action.

What did he mean 'Action'? I hadn't been still for a single second since entering the cage. I had been dodging around trying to keep the bird lady between me and potential death and at the same time trying to interview her. As we talked she kept the condor at bay by feeding it pieces of meat from her leather pouch.

I can't remember a single question or answer in the chaotic time that followed, but if you can imagine the bird eventually getting its head inside the now-empty pouch and then tearing it from the bird lady's shoulder, you will perhaps excuse my lapse of memory. In a moment of foolish bravado, I attempted to recover the pouch and, believe it or not, ended up having a tug of war with this ferocious feathered beast!

Later when, thankful to be out of the cage, I was enjoying a well-earned cup of tea in the centre's canteen, an old man who cleaned the cages out confided another danger to me.

'Listen Mr Vet,' he said, in a suitably respectful tone of voice, leaning forward to add impact to his words of wisdom, 'you got to watch that big bugger,' he said with real feeling. 'Not only can he rip your face off with that beak of his, but only a couple of weeks ago he shat all over me from a great height!'

'Is that right,' I responded, shaking my head sympathetically, and thanking my lucky stars that I hadn't now conducted the interview with the condor circling overhead!

Chapter 14

Fame at Last

The South London street was remarkably quiet, even for seven-thirty in the morning. So much so, that the two Arab gentlemen coming towards me could clearly be seen to be a little excited. I checked to see that my fly wasn't undone and edged out towards the kerb side of the pavement to increase the separation between us slightly when we passed.

When they got within a pace or two from me, they both gave a series of humble little nods and smiling self-consciously greeted me with 'Good morning, Mr Sharif'.

So what I thought might be a threatening situation turned out to be a simple case of mistaken identity. It was not the first time I had been taken for that famous film star, Omar Sharif.

The trouble, now, was that I couldn't return their very friendly greeting because my Scottish accent would have been a dead give-away. I conjured up a weak smile and half lifted a hand to my forehead in response. Somehow this gesture felt a bit more 'Arabic' in nature. In any case I reckoned my raised hand might help hide my blue eyes and the fact that I had no gap between my front teeth!

I hurried on, not daring to look back, and cursed the fact that I hadn't recalled the classic Arab greeting of 'Salam Alykum!' which one of my very own clients had taught me back in my wee surgery in Horsforth.

This client originally came from Baghdad and was the proud owner of a lovely little budgie called Whisky. I remember wondering, at our first meeting, if the teaching of Islam, with its preaching of abstinence would have approved of her choice of name.

Over the years I grew almost as fond of that little bird as Mrs Khammo and her daughter were and indeed it was an exceptional animal. In response to their constant attention Whisky became so tame that he always arrived at the consulting room, not in a cage but proudly perched upon his owner's finger! Among the barking dogs and potentially predatory cats of a vet's surgery, this was quite an impressive trick. Had this been Whisky's only claim to fame I might not have remembered him so vividly. His owner, however, was at pains to tell me that he had other exceptional qualities.

'His favourite trick,' said Mrs Khammo, 'is to lie on his back and push a miniature barbell up and down with his feet.'

My look of surprise was enough to evoke confirmation from Mrs Khammo.

'He does honestly, Meester Baxter. Next time I come, I will show you.'

'I can't wait, Mrs Khammo,' I said, showing her out and trying to picture a budgie 'pumping iron'!

The budgie's next appointment came round more quickly than expected and my first clue that Whisky was in the waiting room was when another client announced it. Clutching a baby in one arm, and a cat basket in the other she burst red-faced into the consulting room.

'What's wrong, Mrs Robinson?' I asked, before getting round to the cat's problem. I could see she was in a bit of a state.

'You won't believe this, Mr Baxter, but there is a foreign lady out there,' she nodded towards the closed waiting-room door, 'and she's got a budgie perched on her finger.'

'Oh yes,' I replied, 'that's Mrs Khammo. 'It's a lovely bird,' I added, just in case Whisky had blotted his copy book and bitten the baby.

'I know that,' retorted Mrs Robinson, eager to get to the point, 'but you know what it did?' I could hardly wait. 'Well,' she said, 'it cocked its little head to one side, looked down at my baby and clear as a bell said "It's a baby!" She shook her head in amazement and repeated ' "It's a baby" – isn't that brilliant? I never knew birds could be that clever.' She was obviously very impressed by the budgie's intelligent appreciation of her offspring!

After I had attended to the lady's cat and sent her and the baby on their way, I ushered in Mrs Khammo with Whisky, as usual, perched on her finger. I recounted the story of the previous client who had been amazed by Whisky's recognition of her baby.

It took a few minutes for the penny to drop but eventually Mrs Khammo managed to work things out. Apparently she and her daughter had both been accustomed to talking to the bird in their own language and one of their favourite phrases was, in common with many British budgie owners, 'I love you...I love you'. This translated into Arabic is '*enta habiby*'. This was what little Whisky had been repeating in the waiting room. So '*enta habiby*' had been understandably misinterpreted as 'it's a baby'! I could just see Mrs Robinson going round her friends recounting the tale of that wonderfully intelligent bird, when in truth it was a misunderstood foreign declaration of love!

Even this unusual episode, however, hadn't made me forget Mrs Khammo's promise to have Whisky do his barbell performance for me and, true to her word, she had brought the equipment with her.

Delving into her bag with her free hand she produced a miniature barbell fashioned out of balsa wood and about three inches long. Placing this on the table she plucked Whisky from her finger and gently positioned him on his back, talking to him all the time.

'Now Whisky, be a good boy for Meester Baxter...*enta habiby*.' Whisky, unbelievably, lay there in this most unlikely position for any bird that still had breath in its body, and awaited the next stage in the act. Picking up the barbell in the tips of the fingers of both hands, she delicately positioned it in Whisky's claws so that he grasped it right in the middle. It was much like being upside down on a wooden perch. Encouraged by Mrs Khammo, Whisky set off at great speed, lifting and lowering the barbell about ten times in quick succession.

'Good boy', applauded Mrs Khammo as Whisky, in a final flourish, threw the barbell from his grasp and then lightly skipped back onto his owner's extended finger!

I was as impressed as Mrs Robinson had been, and I could also see how Whisky might be just the bird to star on 'It's a Vet's Life'.

As I have already mentioned, I had on several occasions been compared in looks to Omar Sharif, so I thought it might be appropriate to borrow the traditional Arab headgear and begin the spot with a very civilized Salam Alykum! After all, the producer said that I should try to please every possible fraction of the potential audience and there were a lot of Arabic-speaking viewers out there. Fortunately, Mr Khammo was only too happy to lend me his *agal wa kafia* and teach me how to wear it!

With the cloth on my head held in place by a round black *agal*, I looked even more like Omar Sharif, but on the producer's advice I decided not to labour the point!

'I think we've got impact enough, John,' he said dryly, 'with you dressed as an Arab sheikh and a budgie who can do a work-out with a barbell!'

Over the years I have been mistaken for many celebrities and to be honest this has been more pleasurable than troublesome. Everyone wants to be attractive to others and even if the attention comes second-hand, it can still be very flattering. Even the reflected glory that comes from being associated with famous people can be pleasurable.

In one of the earlier series of 'It's a Vet's Life' we introduced a celebrity spot to give the programmes a bit of stature and as well as discovering that these stars are just human beings too, I managed to get an insight into some of their 'behind the scenes' personalities.

Geoff Hughes, who at that time was a regular on 'Coronation Street' but who now stars as Orwell in 'Keeping Up Appearances', came on to one programme to talk about his love for the country life and brought with him a couple of orphaned lambs. It made a great contrast to see this 'rough lad from the street' gently feeding a little lamb with a bottle. Tippi Hedren, a Seventies star of the big screen, came on the programme to talk about her home in Africa with a house full of lions, and Ted Rogers, the host of a popular game show called '3-2-1', brought on his wee Yorkie and we discussed the dog's problems instead of talking about Ted.

One of my favourite celebrities was a captivating old Yorkshire lady called Hannah, who had had fame thrust upon her when television producer Barry Cockroft 'discovered' her. He did a documentary on her hard life, running a small hill farm single-handed in the bleak winter countryside of the Dales.

I was grateful that the 'It's a Vet's Life' producer chose a warm summer's day for me to visit Hannah Hawkswell, when I found myself up on her farm interviewing her as she milked one of her old cows.

Because of the success of 'It's a Vet's Life', I had become a bit of a celebrity myself, and requests for personal appearances came flooding in from all quarters. I was asked to open this or that event, or talk to some group or other. The tragedy, of course, is that the more famous you become, the less time you have to do such things. I was not only trying to make more television programmes, but also running a busy veterinary practice! Nevertheless, I did manage to make it to a few of the summer shows, and the agricultural show at Brigg was one of the more memorable.

'We've got a nice car for you to drive round in,' the chairman told me on the phone. 'And, if you don't mind doing a bit of a tour of the exhibits and perhaps presenting some of the prizes, I'm sure that the crowd will love it.'

Still a bit unaccustomed to this star treatment, I arrived at the showground not knowing quite what to expect. My delegated guide from the show committee whisked me away to the chairman's tent for a cup of tea 'or something stronger' and a bit of briefing on my duties.

'The car should be here any minute,' said the chairman. 'Are you sure that you don't want something stronger than that tea?'

I guessed by the flush in his cheeks and the sparkle in his eye that he had already partaken. 'Later,' I parried, 'I'll maybe take a dram after the event.'

'It's here,' announced an unknown head poking round the flap of the tent.

'That will be the car,' translated the chairman. So saying, he and his lady arose and I followed on behind them, in some trepidation. Just outside the tent entrance, resplendent in uniform, cap and polished leather boots, stood an immaculate chauffeur holding open the rear door of an impressive pink Packard convertible. Mrs Chairman smiled her delight and climbed in.

'Okay, John,' said Mr Chairman. 'You are next.' I tried to emulate his wife's beaming face as I climbed in behind her. As her husband clunked the door shut behind him, he had a brainwave.

'I think that it would be a good idea, John, if you were to sit up on the back of the seat, so that the crowd could see you.'

'Okay then,' I said, as if it were all in a day's work for a 'star' like me, and clambered up.

The chauffeur, now in the driving seat, looked over his shoulder. 'Are we ready for the off then?' he asked. The chairman looked at me, smiled and gave him his nod of approval.

So this is show business, I thought silently to myself, as we set off at a steady five miles an hour. Here I was, propped up on the back seat of a big fancy American car...A star! I felt such a fool!

As we reached the first of the multitude of people who thronged around the perimeter of the main ring, I could see them nudge each other in anticipation. In the insecurity of my new-found stardom, I wondered if anyone would even recognize me.

Instead of 'Who is it?' I heard them say, 'It's that vet off t' telly! It's John Baxter.'

One little plump lady clutching a compact camera, pointed it towards me and clicked the shutter. I waved at her, more in gratitude than gracious response. She waved back enthusiastically, and I heard her say as she looked round at her husband, 'Ehh! Isn't he lovely.' Her husband grunted, not at all impressed.

It was as if this lady's fervour had acted as the fuse to a powder keg, and despite our slow progress, the cheering, waving and picture-

Being a guest on Russell Grant's 'Star Choice' programme, with real stars like Katie Boyle and Russell himself, was not only a privilege but a great pleasure.

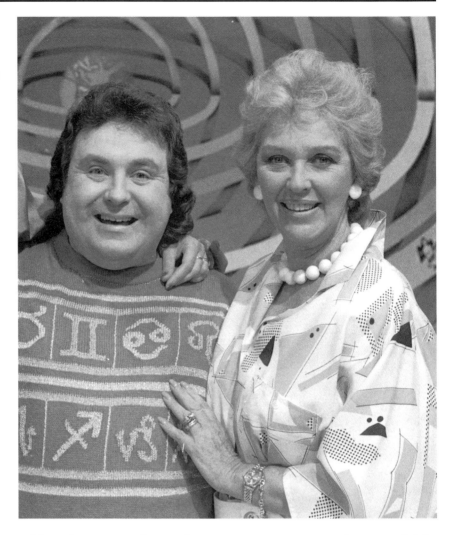

taking throng made my journey seem over much too quickly. Flushed with my unexpected success, I almost sprang from my peacock position when the car stopped. Mr and Mrs Chairman, now both beaming at the crowd's ecstatic response, led me across the green turf of the showground to the VIP tent. As we passed through a small group of 'fans' who had gathered at its entrance, one old lady grabbed my arm as I passed and said in a hushed and reverent tone, 'That's a lovely car you've got, Mr Baxter.'

'Thanks, darling,' I said, not wishing to destroy her illusion that spectacular pink cars were just one of the trappings of stardom!

During the course of the day, what with the shaking of innumerable hands, posing for pictures and signing hundreds of autographs, I got my first glimpse of what 'the glare of limelight' can mean. As the afternoon drew to a close, I was called upon to present the prizes. Handshakes, smiles and silver cups were the order of the day. For the winning ladies' tug of war team there had to be that little extra award, and they decided it should be a cuddle and a kiss from the 'star of the show'.

As I drove home that evening in my own more conservative car, I had a good feeling about the whole affair. Even the painful bruising of my ribs seemed strangely pleasurable. After all, I told myself, those tug of war team ladies had been a bit too big to refuse.

Over the years, as my skills of presenting my own programme grew, I was approached by producers of other shows to perform as a guest. They knew that I and people like me have two things in our favour. We can be depended upon to deliver the goods and our faces are already known on the box.

On one such programme, which was based on astrology, I appeared with Russell Grant. He presided over two amateur teams of astrologers, as they questioned the celebrities, myself included, and tried to ascertain the sign we were all born under. For Russell, 'my blue eyes said everything', and eventually, all were agreed that I was a Scorpio.

For me, the programme was an enjoyable experience, but the after-show meal came as a bit of a mixed blessing. Russell himself was charming and hungry all the way through, but one guest celebrity seemed to dislike me from the moment my astrological sign was ascertained. In the taxi on the way to the restaurant, she mumbled something about her father being a Scorpio, and proclaimed that although I appeared outwardly pleasant, she knew I was not so nice under the surface! I never did find out why she so disliked Scorpios, but since our paths were unlikely to cross again, it didn't seriously worry me.

Katie Boyle, on the other hand, thought that I was quite wonderful. Not, I may say, for any personal quality that I possessed, but simply because I was a vet and, therefore, likely to be an animal-lover like herself.

Since then, I have made numerous guest appearances on many other programmes, like 'This Morning' with Judy Finnigan and Richard Madeley, where I learned a lot about the skills needed in live television. Not the least of these is the ability to think on the spot as viewers phone in live questions and expect sensible answers.

Appearing on other television programmes is, of course, good publicity for 'It's a Vet's Life' and for that very purpose I agreed to make the long journey from Yorkshire to Southampton to appear on 'TV Weekly' with Eamonn Holmes.

The programme researcher was good enough to book me flights from Leeds Bradford to Southampton airport and then the plan was to take me to Heathrow by car after the show and from there fly me back home. As my own show was currently enjoying a seventeen-week series on ITV, the publicity would be welcome, so it seemed like a good idea all round. Then the snow started, and it didn't stop. The airports closed and I was forced to change my arrangements and travel by train. I left home at seven in the morning and got home at nine at night. My total time on screen was four minutes! It wasn't easy explaining to my clients the next day why such a short appearance on the telly can be so tiring.

Where your 'fame' or 'celebrity status' really shows is out on the street. If you are recognizable, but not instantly so, it is often sufficient to keep walking and to avoid actual eye-contact with anyone. If you do this, it is only children or a few 'mentally-challenged' adults who have the bravado to grab your passing arm or poke a knowing finger in your face.

If you stop, or are stopped, the public have time to place you and if one of them should decide to mark the occasion by requesting an autograph you could be in big trouble! Even the lowliest of 'celebrities' can collect quite a crowd in next to no time! Of course the television companies are aware of this public desire for contact with anyone who has been on the box and will generally have furnished their stars with an ample supply of presigned publicity pictures. The trouble is that many celebrities are quite shy when not working and may be nothing at all like their on-screen personality.

James Herriot, the eminent vet and author, has experienced world fame but doesn't like the media attention his prominence has attracted. He told me that his book-publicizing tours of America were so arduous that he would be most unwilling to repeat them. In real life there could be no nicer man, but he confesses that he finds it very difficult to deal with the public attention that his success has brought with it. Before he retired from practising as a vet, he even had to set aside one afternoon a week to accommodate visiting Americans who had crossed the Atlantic to meet him.

In one of the earlier series of 'It's a Vet's Life', the producer decided to run a competition in conjunction with the programme, to name two little puppies who had featured in the show. One of the prizes suggested was to be a James Herriot book autographed by the author himself. Since I knew him personally I volunteered to make the journey to Thirsk for that purpose. So, having loaded a cardboard box containing a dozen copies of the compendium edition of his books, I set off along the A1.

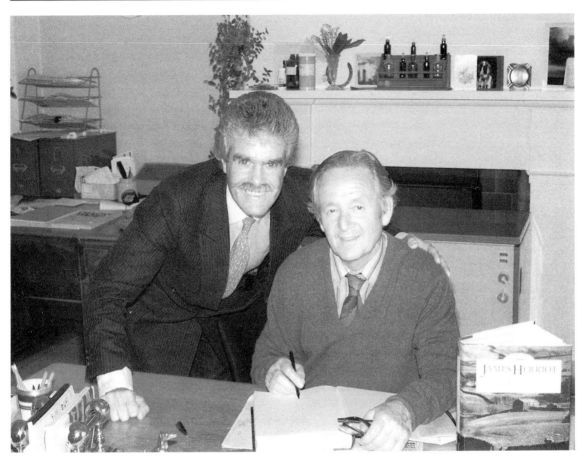

The world's most famous vet, James Herriot, signs some copies of his book. These became much sought-after prizes in a competition on 'It's a Vet's Life'.

It was a pleasant summer's day and as I drove up, with my elbow leaning on the open car window, I looked forward to my pre-arranged meeting with James Herriot. I glanced over my shoulder at the box on the back seat, which had just come from the booksellers that very morning, and mused on the colossal achievement of the man.

I hope they have given me the right books, I said to myself thoughtfully. No good arriving at Thirsk and pulling out another author's books for the great James Herriot to sign. As my concern fed on itself, I felt compelled to check and, trying to keep my eyes on the road, I stretched back with one hand and tore open the top of the box. It was then that everything went white rather than black! Unknown to me the books had been packed in those white polystyrene pieces, and when the rush of air from the open window caught them, it blew them around the car interior like a miniature snowstorm! Through the swirling white flakes I could just discern the bemused faces of drivers heading in the other direction. I guess my car must have looked a bit like one of those snowflake-filled glass ornaments that children love so much at Christmas! I hurriedly wound up the window and the 'snowstorm' subsided.

Despite this near catastrophe, I arrived safely at James Herriot's practice and struggled into the surgery with my box of books. It was then that a better idea occurred to me. What if I got the famous author's picture as well as his autograph on the books? That really would be a prize worth having!

Fortunately a visiting pharmaceutical representative agreed to take the picture as I posed at the shoulder of James Herriot while he signed his name on the flyleaf.

'What do you want with such a picture, John?' he asked, looking up at me.

'Well, Alf,' I replied, using his real name 'I could always say that here was a picture of the most famous vet in the world...' I hesitated then continued, 'and another!'

Alf looked thoughtful for a moment, then with a twinkle in his eye and showing the genuine niceness of a truly great man he retorted 'Aye John, but which one am I?'

I still have one of those pictures to this day and it hangs proudly on the wall of my own surgery.

True stature is, of course, given to very few and can be remarkably durable. The transient variety which is often held by those who know only fleeting fame on the telly can be demolished by the unlikeliest of contacts.

One weekend I was enjoying a pleasant break with my wife Alice in Blackpool when I noticed a lone middle-aged gentleman approaching us on the esplanade. The light in his eyes and the smile of recognition on his face told me instantly that he was a 'fan'. I prepared myself for a friendly 'Hello. How are you?' as I walked on by.

Stopping squarely in front of me he stymied my plan and thrusting out a hand, announced in a loud voice, 'I know you. You're Derek Batey!'

My smile momentarily faded at this unintended error. Not that there was anything wrong with Derek Batey. In fact he was a very popular and handsome man who presented a television show called 'Mr and Mrs', but the only similarity I could see between us was the grey colour of our hair!

'No. No!' I said, rekindling a full-blooded smile, 'I'm not Derek Batey, I'm...' The gentleman, unswayed by my protestations, cut me short.

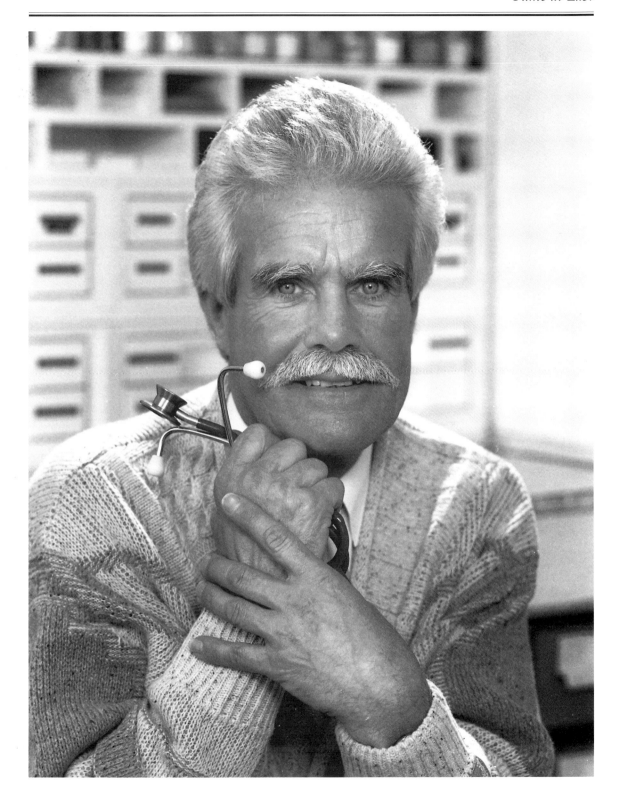

'Give me your autograph, Derek,' he insisted, 'my wife will never believe I've met you.'

'Have one of these,' I said, pulling a coloured publicity picture from my inside pocket. 'What is your name?' I asked, clicking my pen into readiness.

'Albert,' he replied, 'Mr Albert...'

'I'll just put Albert,' I interrupted him, 'it's more personal.' 'With best wishes to Albert' I wrote and very legibly added 'from John Baxter'.

Albert fairly snatched the picture from my hand and scrutinized it avidly. Then he looked up into my eyes and, with a knowing smile, said 'I knew you were Derek Batey!' then marched off down the esplanade clutching his prize.